Simplified
Chair Yoga

for Seniors Over 60

A 25-Day Guides for All Levels to Achieve Better Posture bliss, Mobility, Heart Health, and Weight Loss in 10 Minutes Daily

Coach Dave Francis

<u>About The Author: Coach Dave Francis</u>

Coach Dave Francis is a seasoned wellness advocate and a prominent authority in chair yoga, dedicating over two decades to redefine fitness for seniors. His passion for holistic health evolved into a specialization in adapting traditional yoga practices, culminating in the creation of the transformative "Simplified Chair Yoga for Seniors Over 60: A 25-Day Guides for All Levels." Beyond physical exercise, Coach Dave seamlessly integrates mindfulness, cardiac health, flexibility, and weight management into each session, offering a comprehensive pathway to well-being. His warm coaching approach resonates with practitioners, instilling confidence and encouragement, making wellness an inclusive and pleasurable journey for all.

Introduction:

Elevate Your Well-Being Through Chair Yoga

Welcome to an exciting and transforming adventure designed just for the dynamic group of seniors aged 60 and over. "Chair Yoga Unlocked" is more than a book; it's a rejuvenation blueprint, a key to unlocking the door to a life full of energy, strength, and overall wellbeing.

The Health and Age Tapestry

Our bodies' intricate demands evolve in tandem with the passage of time. What was simple before now demands focus and care. The beauty of chair yoga is that it is an elegant combination of old wisdom and modern adaptation, custom-crafted to fit the particular needs of seniors navigating their health path.

Chair Yoga: From Mysterious to Mastery

Yoga frequently evokes images of twisted poses on mats, which may appear intimidating or impractical to many seniors. "Chair Yoga Unlocked" on the other hand highlights the route to comprehensive wellbeing via a practice that is strongly rooted in accessibility and comfort. It provides a new viewpoint on yoga, demystifying it by putting it into the ease of a sitting practice.

Breaking Down Barriers and Promoting Empowerment

Consider a world in which skepticism fades, physical restrictions become opportunities, and temporal constraints become doable routines. This is the core of "Chair Yoga Unlocked" – a thorough handbook aimed to empower as much as inform. It talks straight to the heart, guaranteeing that there are no obstacles to wellbeing and that age is only a number in the pursuit of life.

Beyond Posture: A Journey to Wholeness

Explore chapters that go beyond the physical realm to delve into the depths of wellbeing. Each aspect of "Chair Yoga Unlocked" is precisely intended to restore balance and energize the mind, body, and soul, from breathing exercises that refresh to positions that redefine mobility and meditations that feed the spirit.

The 25-Day Transformation Journey

A highly designed 25-day program, precisely calibrated to accommodate all levels of fitness and skill, is at the heart of this voyage. Begin your journey through beginner, intermediate, and advanced challenges, with each step guiding you toward better posture, increased mobility, heart health, and weight control. Every day brings the prospect of a renewed sense of well-being.

A Vibrant Way of Life Awaits

"Chair Yoga Unlocked" does not stop at the covers; it extends an invitation to embrace a wellness-enriched existence. It invites you to incorporate mindfulness into your everyday activities, cultivating an energy that emanates from a holistic approach to wellness.

Your invitation is on its way.

This isn't simply a book for seniors over 60; it's your personal invitation to go on a revolutionary adventure. Accept this chance to improve your posture, improve your heart health, lose weight, and live a more vibrant life. "Chair Yoga Unlocked" is more than just a book; it's a companion on your road to a better, happier self.

Chapter 1: The Essence of Yoga

Welcome to an enlightening journey through a practice that spans ages, countries, and borders – welcome to the enthralling world of yoga. We will peel back the layers of time to grasp the profound roots and essence of yoga, an ancient practice that continues to weave its transformational power into the fabric of our lives.

The Ancient Origins of Yoga

Yoga has been practiced for thousands of years and originated in ancient India. Its origins may be traced back to the Vedas, ancient writings that revealed spiritual teachings and rituals. References to yogic concepts, contemplative techniques, and spiritual ceremonies appear throughout these ancient books, setting the groundwork for what would grow into the diverse practice we know today.

The Legacy of Sage Patanjali: The Birth of Classical Yoga

Patanjali, a guru who lived around 2,000 years ago, published the "Yoga Sutras," a key treatise that defined the intellectual and practical parts of yoga. The eight limbs of yoga are contained within these sutras, providing a complete framework spanning moral norms, postures (asanas), breath control (pranayama), concentration, meditation, and the attainment of spiritual enlightenment (Samadhi). Patanjali's work acts as a beacon of light, illuminating the road to self-realization and transcendence.

Yoga's Cross-Continent Journey: Influences and Diversification

Yoga spread throughout continents over millennia, encountering many civilizations and evolving into numerous forms. From medieval India's Hatha Yoga scriptures, which emphasized physical postures and breath control, to Tantra Yoga, which explored the union of opposites, and Bhakti Yoga, which cultivated devotion, each school enhanced yoga's tapestry, adding hues of spirituality, physicality, and awareness.

Global Resurgence and Adaptations of Yoga in the Modern Era

Yoga experienced a renaissance in the twentieth century, crossing geographical boundaries and capturing the attention of the Western world. Yoga was brought to the West by pioneers such as Swami Vivekananda and Paramahansa Yogananda, who sparked interest in its comprehensive advantages. As interest grew, new yoga styles arose, ranging from the vigorous Vinyasa flow to the meditative Yin Yoga, to meet a wide range of preferences and requirements.

Yoga's Essence: Beyond the Physical Practice

Yoga, at its essence, transcends the physical postures that are commonly associated with it. It's a symbiotic union of mind, body, and spirit – a comprehensive way of living that fosters self-awareness, inner calm, and alignment with global consciousness. Yoga acts as a beacon beyond the mat, directing practitioners toward unification, balance, and a profound connection with themselves and the world around them.

Embracing Timeless Wisdom in Yoga: A Call to Transformation

We discover a treasure mine of wisdom as we unravel the historical fabric of yoga, a legacy passed down through millennia. This ancient discipline invites us to go on a transforming journey that transcends materiality to find our real essence – a voyage of self-discovery, balance, and profound inner serenity.

Discovering the principles and different types of yoga practice

Welcome to a journey beyond physical movement, a journey into the timeless principles and multifarious practices of yoga. We'll study the different tapestry of yoga techniques, each offering a unique road towards holistic well-being and self-discovery as we navigate the depths of this ancient practice.

The Yogic Wisdom Pillars: Unveiling the Principles

The core principles of yoga act as guiding lights on the path to self-realization and enlightenment. These ancient wisdom-based ideas are the foundation of a holistic lifestyle:

- *Ahimsa (Nonviolence):* Accepting compassion and not injuring oneself or others.

- Satya (Honesty): Accepting honesty and sincerity in one's ideas, words, and actions.

- *Asteya (non-stealing):* Developing integrity and non-covetous thinking.

- *Brahmacharya (Moderation):* Adopting self-control and a balanced way of life.

- *Aparigraha (Non-attachment):* Releasing possessiveness and embracing detachment.

Yoga's Spectrum: Diverse Paths to Harmony

- **Hatha Yoga:** is the fundamental discipline of yoga that focuses on physical postures (asanas) and breath control (pranayama). It's a simple technique that promotes strength, flexibility, and relaxation.

- **Vinyasa Yoga:** is a dynamic practice that synchronizes movement with breath and flows through sequences that improve strength, agility, and awareness.

- **Iyengar Yoga:** The hallmarks of this approach are precision and alignment, with props used to support asanas and encourage safe, deep stretching.

- **Kundalini Yoga:** A type of yoga that focuses on breathwork, chanting, and certain postures to awaken spiritual energy (kundalini) and create inner transformation.

- **Ashtanga Yoga** is a systematic and intense practice that consists of a set of postures performed in a prescribed sequence to promote strength, flexibility, and focus.

- **Bikram/Hot Yoga:** This practice is performed in a heated room and follows a specified sequence of 26 postures and two breathing exercises that promote detoxification and flexibility.

- **Yin Yoga:** is a slow-paced practice that focuses on connective tissues by maintaining poses for prolonged periods of time to increase flexibility and induce relaxation.

- **Restorative Yoga:** Using props for support, this practice strives to fully relax the body, allowing for healing and renewal.

- **Jivamukti Yoga** is a practice that combines physical postures, chanting, meditation, and ethical precepts to promote spiritual growth and social activity.

- **Yoga Nidra:** Also known as "yogic sleep," this practice promotes inner calm and healing by inducing profound relaxation and meditation.

Beyond Physical Postures: Uncovering the Essence

Beyond the many kinds of yoga, there is a common element – the unification of mind, body, and spirit. While asanas are a physical part of yoga, the practice invites practitioners to explore meditation, breathwork, and awareness. Each style provides a distinct path to this unity, leading to a greater awareness of oneself and the connectivity of the cosmos.

What is Chair Yoga: Its Nature, Accessibility, and Universal Benefits

Welcome to the world of Chair Yoga, a transforming experience that pushes the boundaries of yoga. As we engage on this journey, we'll discover the nature, accessibility, and deep advantages that make Chair Yoga a gateway to overall well-being for people of all ages and physical abilities.

Understanding Chair Yoga: A Seated Wellness Path

Chair Yoga is a harmonic combination of conventional yoga concepts modified to assist practitioners who may have mobility, flexibility, or balance issues. It incorporates the essence of yoga through a sitting practice, integrating modified postures and gentle movements performed while seated or with the use of a chair.

The Accessibility of the Chair Yoga

One of Chair Yoga's distinguishing characteristics is its extraordinary accessibility. It removes the restrictions that conventional yoga may have, making the practice accessible to elders, people with physical impairments, office workers looking for lunchtime relaxation, and anybody looking for a light start to yoga. Its versatility allows it to accept everyone, regardless of age or fitness level.

The Universal benefits of the Chair Yoga

1. **Enhanced Flexibility:** Chair Yoga stretches and mobilizes joints gently, creating flexibility without the pressure of floor-based poses.
2. **Improvesd posture:** Chair Yoga works in straightening the spine and strengthening core muscles, promoting better posture, via mindful movements and sitting positions.
3. **Stress Reduction:** Chair Yoga incorporates mindful breathing exercises and relaxation methods to reduce stress and promote mental clarity and relaxation.

4. **Increased Mobility:** Gentle motions help to improve range of motion, resulting in improved functional mobility for daily tasks.

5. **Strengthening Muscles:** Chair Yoga uses body weight and resistance to build muscles and improve overall physical strength.

6. **balancing Improvement:** Modified balancing postures performed with the assistance of a chair or against a wall increase stability and balance.

7. **Mental Clarity:** Using mindfulness and breathing practices together cultivates mental concentration and tranquillity, lowering anxiety and boosting general well-being.

The Seated Poses and Modified Movements

- *Seated Mountain Pose (Tadasana):* A grounding and aligning posture that promotes awareness and stability when seated.

- *Seated Cat-Cow Stretch:* Promotes spinal flexibility and stress relief with moderate motions.
- *Chair Warrior postures:* Modified warrior postures that improve strength and balance while sitting.
- *Seated Twist (Ardha Matsyendrasana):* Promotes spinal mobility and digestion with mild twisting motions.
- *Chair Pigeon Pose:* This stretch stretches the hip muscles to relieve stress and enhance hip flexibility.
- *Mindful Breathing Techniques:* Using pranayama (breathwork) to relax, focus, and reduce stress.

Incorporating Chair Yoga into Daily Life to Increase Accessibility

The appeal of Chair Yoga is its applicability to a variety of venues. A chair may be found in a variety of settings, including offices, community centers, retirement homes, and even the comfort of one's own home. Its adaptability invites you to weave yoga into the fabric of your everyday routines, promoting moments of renewal in the midst of life's demands.

Chair Yoga Remedy for Specific Injuries

Welcome to the world of Chair Yoga's therapeutic brilliance, where the soft embrace of yoga meets the intricacies of injury healing. This investigation will reveal how Chair Yoga functions as a healing sanctuary, providing specialized practices to ease discomfort and help in rehabilitation for certain conditions.

Understanding Chair Yoga's Approach to Harnessing the Healing Power

Chair Yoga is a therapeutic paradise, with its sat postures, reduced movements, and mindfulness practices. Because of its versatility, it is an excellent practice for those negotiating the intricacies of injury rehabilitation. Chair Yoga, by stressing gentle stretches, regulated movements, and attentive breathing, becomes a healing channel, aiding rehabilitation while respecting the body's limits.

Customized Treatments: Chair Yoga for Specific Injuries

Note: Always contact a healthcare practitioner before beginning any fitness plan, especially if you are recuperating from an injury. The following are generic guidelines that should be changed depending on individual requirements and guidance.

1. Lower Back Pain:

    - *Seated Forward Fold:* Gentle forward bends help to stretch and relax the lower back muscles.

    - *Seated Cat-Cow Stretch:* Promotes flexibility and relieves back pain by encouraging mild spinal movement.

2. Knee Injuries:

    - *Seated Leg Extensions:* These exercises strengthen the quadriceps and improve knee mobility without putting strain on the joint.

    - *Chair Warrior Poses:* Modified variations aid in the development of leg strength and stability.

3. Shoulder Problems:

- *Stretching and expanding the shoulders,* alleviating tension and enhancing flexibility with seated Eagle Arms.
- *Seated Shoulder Rolls:* These exercises promote mobility and reduce stiffness in the shoulders and upper back.

4. Arthritis:

- *Seated Twists:* Gentle twists enhance spinal mobility, which aids in the reduction of stiffness and pain.
- *Mindful Breathing Exercises:* Promotes relaxation, reduces tension, and alleviates arthritic symptoms.

5. Sciatica:

- *Seated Pigeon Pose:* Reduces sciatic nerve irritation by relieving tension in the hips and lower back.
- *Seated Side Stretches:* Reduces hip and lower back tension, providing relief from sciatic discomfort.

While Chair Yoga's customized practices target specific ailments, its holistic nature promotes mental and emotional well-being, both of which are important parts of the healing process:

1. *Stress Reduction:* Mindful breathing and relaxation practices reduce stress, fostering a healing atmosphere.
2. *Improved Circulation:* Gentle motions increase blood flow, which aids in the healing of injuries.
3. *Increased Flexibility:* Gentle stretches increase range of motion, which aids in injury rehabilitation and reduces stiffness.
4. *strength-building:* postures help to restore muscle strength without stressing affected regions.
5. *Emotional Support:* The mindfulness of Chair Yoga promotes a positive outlook, which is vital for coping with the hardships of injury rehabilitation.

Principles to follow: Adaptation and Safety

Chair Yoga adaptation for individual ailments necessitates focus and prudence. Always put safety first and pay attention to your body. Modify postures as required, avoid movements that cause discomfort, and seek individualized modifications from a trained teacher or healthcare expert.

YOGA EXCERCISES

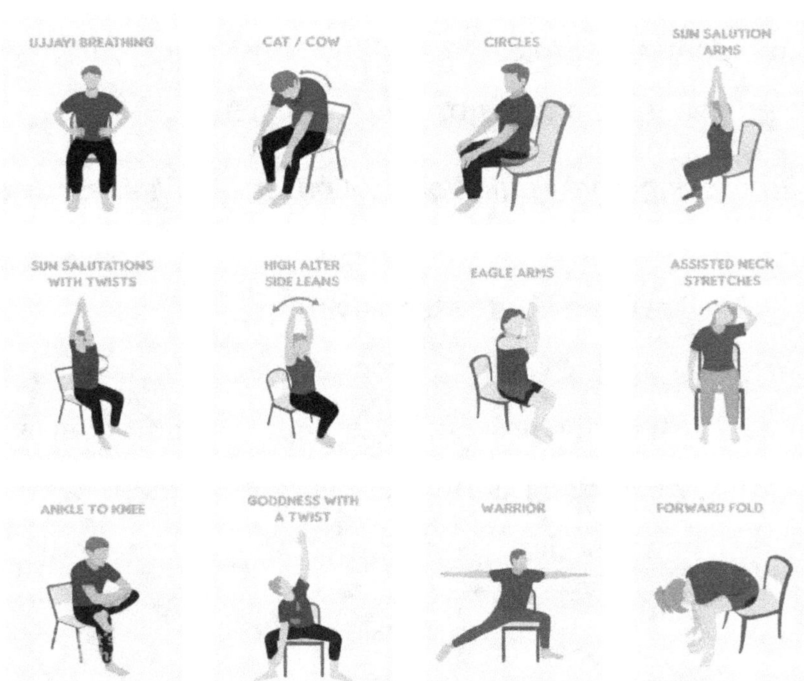

Chapter 2: Preparing for Chair Yoga Journey

Possessing the Right Mindset for a Fulfilling Chair Yoga Experience

Welcome to the beginning of your Chair Yoga adventure! Before diving into the physical postures and gentle motions, it's critical to build the proper attitude – a mindset that sets the scene for a rewarding and enlightening Chair Yoga adventure. In this chapter, we'll look at the importance of mental preparation, overcoming typical hurdles, ensuring safety, and preparing for a transforming experience.

Embracing the Chair Yoga Mindset: A Wellness Mental Canvas

1. Openness and responsiveness:
   Chair Yoga encourages openness and responsiveness to adaptations and variations. Accept the notion that every movement, no matter how modest, contributes to your overall well-being.

2. Patience and compassion:

    Train yourself to be patient with yourself. Chair
    Yoga is about growth, not perfection. Approach
    each session with care for yourself, respecting
    your body's particular talents and limits.

3. Chair Yoga relies heavily on attention and
    presence.

    Allow yourself to fully feel the exercise by being
    present in each movement and breath. Allow
    distractions to leave and accept the calm of the
    present.

4. Gratitude and Self-Care:

    Consider Chair Yoga to be a kind of self-care.
    Cultivate gratitude for your body's talents by
    engaging in a nurturing and revitalizing activity.

Overcoming Common Obstacles: Making Room

- *Physical Restrictions:* Chair Yoga is designed
  specifically for people who have physical
  restrictions. Accept adaptations and variations
  that meet the demands of your body, ensuring
  a safe and comfortable practice.

- *Self-doubt and Expectations:* Let go of your ideas about what Chair Yoga should look like. Every practice is unique; instead of comparing to preconceived ideas, concentrate on the feelings and advantages.

- *Time Restriction:* Chair Yoga works with your schedule. Even a few minutes each day can have a huge impact. Consistency should take precedence over duration.

- *Lack of Space or Equipment:* Chair Yoga takes little more than a chair and your commitment. It's a simple technique that overcomes physical limitations.

Safety First, use caution when doing chair yoga.

1. *Consultation with a Healthcare expert:* Before beginning any new workout regimen, including Chair Yoga, seek guidance from a healthcare expert, especially if you have any current health issues or injuries.

2. *Listening to Your Body:* Pay attention to your body's signals. If a movement causes discomfort or pain, slow down or change your posture. It's often said to stay within what feels comfortable, but stepping outside that zone can lead to growth and new experiences.

3. *Limitation Awareness:* Recognize your limitations and work within your range of motion. You will see growth with time and practice, but never force a movement beyond your body's capabilities.

4. *The Breath as Your Guide:* The breath is central to Chair Yoga. Allow it to guide you; it should flow naturally and comfortably. Avoid holding your breath or straining.

Setting the Scene: Designing Your Chair Yoga Sanctuary

- A calm Area:

  Set aside a calm, clutter-free area for your practice. It doesn't have to be enormous; a comfy nook would suffice.

- comfortable attire:

  Wear loose that allows for free mobility without restraint. Ascertain that your chair is solid and supportive.

- Mindful Preparation:

  Before beginning your practice, spend a few moments in peaceful meditation or deep breathing. Set goals for your session while maintaining a pleasant attitude.

Addressing Common Obstacles and Misconceptions in Yoga Practice

Welcome to a place where we dispel the beliefs and hurdles that may be preventing you from embarking on the transforming path of yoga. As we progress through this inquiry, we'll dispel myths, break down barriers, and provide insights to help you overcome typical roadblocks to a meaningful yoga practice.

1. I'm Not Flexible Enough for Yoga

One of the most common misconceptions about yoga is that flexibility is required. In truth, yoga is a journey toward increasing flexibility, strength, and overall well-being, rather than contorting into pretzel-like positions. Yoga is suitable for people of all body types and levels of flexibility. Flexibility develops over time with constant practice.

Overcoming the Obstacle: Accept adaptations and variations that are customized to your body's requirements. Begin with easy, beginner-friendly courses or styles such as Hatha or Yin Yoga, stressing progress rather than perfection.

2. Some folks think yoga is just for those who are young and already in great shape.

Yoga transcends age, size, and degree of fitness. It's a practice that everyone can do, regardless of age or physical condition. There is a yoga style for everyone, from Chair Yoga for elderly or those with physical disabilities to intense Vinyasa sequences.

Overcoming the Obstacle: Try out several styles and classes until you discover one that speaks to you. Remember that yoga meets you where you are and grows with you.

3. Yoga is religious or spiritual

While yoga has spiritual roots, its current practice does not need religious affiliation. Mindfulness, breathwork, and physical postures that promote health and well-being are at the heart of yoga. It is a welcoming practice available to people of all religions and beliefs.

Overcoming the Obstacle: Accept the components of yoga that speak to you, whether it's the physical practice, mindfulness methods, or breathwork. Yoga has a wide range of advantages that go beyond spirituality.

4. I Don't Have Time for Yoga

Time is frequently perceived as a limited resource in our fast-paced environment. However, even a few minutes of yoga practice every day might have a substantial impact. Yoga fits into your schedule, whether it's a quick morning routine or a noon stretch.

Overcoming the Obstacle: Make your well-being a priority by scheduling little amounts of time for yoga. Even a short period of practice may have a significant influence on your physical and mental wellbeing.

5. Yoga Is Too Expensive

Many people are put off by the idea that yoga is an expensive pastime because of the cost of lessons or equipment. However, yoga does not necessitate the purchase of expensive memberships or equipment. There are a plethora of free or low-cost options accessible online or at community centers.

Overcoming the Challenge: Look for free or low-cost resources, online lessons, community workshops, or simply practice at home with a mat or a basic towel. Yoga does not necessitate exorbitant expenditures in order to gain its advantages

6. I Need to Be Silent or Meditative During Yoga,

contrary to common assumption, does not necessarily necessitate full quiet or a contemplative state. While some practices include meditation or times of solitude, others include movement, music, or instructor instruction. Yoga may be dynamic, allowing for a variety of expressions and energy.

Overcoming the Obstacle: Find a style or class that fits your degree of comfort. Yoga provides a variety of experiences; explore until you discover an atmosphere that meets your needs.

7. I Need to Look a Certain Way to Do Yoga

Images of yoga in the media frequently reflect a certain body type or look. Yoga, on the other hand, is for everyone; it's about how you feel, not how you appear. Accept your individuality and practice without feeling obligated to adhere to stereotypes.

Overcoming the Obstacle: Pay attention to how yoga makes you feel, both mentally and physically. Let go of preconceived notions and accept the practice as a personal path of self-discovery and well-being.

8. Yoga Is Only for Women

While yoga sessions may appear to be dominated by women, yoga is for everyone, regardless of gender. Yoga has no gender-specific advantages, such as enhanced flexibility, strength, mental clarity, and stress reduction.

Overcoming the Obstacle: Accept yoga as a discipline that transcends gender norms. Find a supportive group or class that includes practitioners of both genders, promoting an inclusive environment.

9. I Can't Focus or Quiet My Mind

Many people assume that in order to practice yoga, one must acquire perfect mental calm or tranquility, which can be difficult, especially for beginners. Yoga is about fostering awareness rather than reaching perfect mental silence.

Overcoming the Obstacle: Recognize that a wandering mind is normal. During practice, focus on your breath or the sensations in your body, gently drawing your attention back when distractions emerge.

10. I'm Too Old to Start Yoga

Age should never be an impediment to practicing yoga. Yoga, in fact, may be quite good for seniors, as it promotes flexibility, balance, joint health, and mental well-being. Chair Yoga, mild flows, and restorative practices are appropriate for people of all ages.

Overcoming the Obstacle: Yoga may be practiced at any age. Begin with gentle techniques that are appropriate for your level of comfort and work your way up. Seek for sessions designed exclusively for elders or those looking for a more moderate practice.

11. Yoga Is Just Stretching; It Doesn't Provide a Workout"

Yoga is more than simply stretching; it is a comprehensive practice that includes strength, flexibility, balance, and endurance. Dynamic forms like as Vinyasa or Ashtanga may give a challenging exercise while also improving strength and cardiovascular health.

Overcoming the Obstacle: Experiment with different yoga styles or classes that correspond to your fitness goals. Engage in more dynamic flows or sequences that put your strength and endurance to the test.

12. People might believe they have to be youthful or super fit to start practicing yoga, but that's not the case.

Yoga is suitable for people of various shapes, sizes, and fitness levels. It's a practice that meets you just where you're at. Yoga does not require you to be young or in top physical shape to begin; it adjusts to your demands.

Overcoming the Obstacle: Let rid of the idea that yoga is exclusive for certain body types. Accept yoga as a discipline that promotes diversity and provides benefits to all bodies.

Practical Tips for Ensuring a Safe and Enjoyable Chair Yoga Practice

Welcome to the world of Chair Yoga, where every sat position, every gentle movement, and every focused breath adds to your well-being. We'll uncover practical strategies and insights to promote a safe, rewarding, and joyful Chair Yoga practice, promoting a path toward overall wellbeing and vitality.

Tip 1: Safety and consultation should be prioritized.

- *Consultation with a Healthcare expert:*
  Seek guidance from a certified healthcare expert before beginning any new fitness plan, especially if you are recuperating from an accident or coping with a health problem. Their advice assures your safety and connects your practice with your health requirements.

- *Pay Attention to Your Body:*
  During practice, pay attention to your body's cues. If a movement produces discomfort or suffering, slow down or change your posture. To avoid injury, avoid pushing yourself beyond your comfort zone.

Tip 2: Create a Comfortable and Supportive Environment

- *Select a Stable Chair:*
  Select a solid, stable chair that does not have wheels. Ascertain that it provides enough support

and comfort, letting you to sit with your feet flat on the floor and a neutral spine.

- *Make a Quiet, Safe Space.*

   Designate a clutter-free location with plenty of room for moving. Maintain sufficient lighting and ventilation to create a relaxing and focused environment.

Tip 3: Dress comfortably for movement.

- *Wear Comfortable Clothes:*

   Choose loose, breathable clothes that allows for free mobility. Make sure your clothing does not interfere with your practice or create pain.

- *Consider Footwear:*

   If your practice includes standing poses or movements, use non-slip shoes or go barefoot if it's safe and comfortable for you.

Tip 4: Concentrate on your breathing and mindfulness.

- *Mindful Breathing:* Focus your practice on the breath. Allow your calm, deep breaths to guide your actions. Relax and connect with each position by using the breath.

- *Practice Mindfulness:*
Pay attention to each action and breath. Let rid of distractions, thoughts, and anxieties by focusing your attention on your bodily sensations and the rhythm of your breath.

Tip 5: Begin Slowly and Gradually.

- *Begin with Warm-Ups:*
Begin your practice with easy warm-up movements, stretching, and joint mobilization. Allow your body to wake up and prepare for the upcoming session.

- *Progress Gradually:*
increase your comfort level by attempting deeper stretches or more difficult poses. To minimize strain, constantly respect your body's limits and advance gently.

Tip: Accept Modifications and Variations

- *If necessary, utilize props* :

  such as blocks, blankets, or pillows to assist with your practice. They can help with alignment and make some positions easier to achieve.

- *Modify postures as Needed:*

  Adjust postures to meet the demands of your body. Investigate variants or modified versions of postures to meet any limits or pain.

Tip: Pay Attention to Posture and Alignment

- *Maintain Good Posture:*

  Pay extra attention to appropriate alignment, especially when seated. To support your back, engage your core muscles, relax your shoulders, and maintain your spine erect.

- *Pay Attention to Alignment signals:*

  Pay attention to alignment signals from teachers or reputable sources. Each pose's safety and efficiency are ensured by proper alignment.

Tip 8: Know your limits and take breaks when needed.

- *Respect Your Boundaries:*
  Yoga is not about pushing yourself past your limits. Accept your limitations and avoid comparing your work to that of others. Every person is unique.
- *Take Rest Periods:*
  If you are tired or overwhelmed, take rest periods as required. Resting allows your body to recuperate, which helps to prevent overexertion or damage.

Tip 9: Hydrate and Rehydrate

- *Pre-Practice Hydration:*
  To ensure appropriate hydration, drink water before beginning your practice. If necessary, sip water during breaks, but avoid overconsumption, which may cause pain.
- *Hydration after practice:*
  Rehydrate after practice to recover lost fluids. Pay attention to your body's hydration cues.

Tip 10: Practice Mindful Closure and Relaxation.

- *Mindful Closure:*

  Finish your practice consciously, gently shifting from movement to rest. Take a few seconds to appreciate your practice and its advantages.

- *Relaxation and Savasana:*

  At the end of your practice, give yourself a period of relaxation or a brief Savasana (corpse posture). Resting in quiet integrates your practice's advantages and encourages relaxation

Chair Yoga Safety: What to Avoid During Sessions

Welcome to an investigation that will protect your Chair Yoga journey by steering you clear of potential traps and assuring a practice that promotes your well-being. In this article, we'll look at things to avoid during Chair Yoga sessions in order to maintain a safe, enjoyable, and successful practice that promotes overall wellbeing and vitality.

1. *Avoid excessive exertion or strain.*

   Chair Yoga focuses on slow, deliberate movements and positions. Avoid putting yourself through pain or pressure. Excessive effort might result in muscular strain or damage. Instead, respect your body's boundaries and move slowly within your comfort zone.

2. *Try not to hold your breath.*

   Yoga practice is around mindful breathing. Holding your breath during poses or transitions is not recommended. Instead, keep a natural, rhythmic breath that corresponds to your motions. Holding your breath causes stress and disrupts the flow of energy throughout your body.

3. *Don't force or push yourself over your limits.*

   Resist the impulse to force oneself into an unpleasant or painful stance. Everybody is different, and Chair Yoga allows for adjustments and variations. Respect your limitations and pay attention to your body's cues. Gradually increase your ability without pushing yourself too much.

4. *Do not rely solely on the chair for support.*

While the chair provides stability and support, it should not be relied on excessively or used as a crutch. Instead of relying totally on the chair's support, engage your core muscles and use it as a tool for balance. This aids in the development of strength and stability in your practice.

5. *Avoid making comparisons or making judgments.*

Avoid comparing your skills to those of others or assessing yourself based on perceived talents. Yoga is a personal experience, and each person's practice is unique. During your sessions, embrace your individuality, acknowledge your development, and let go of any judgments or self-criticism.

6. *Take your time with poses and transitions.*

Chair Yoga promotes careful transitions between poses and focused movement. Avoid hastening through postures or transitions. Instead, concentrate on the quality of your motions, synchronizing them with your breath, and remaining mindful throughout the practice.

7.   *Do Not Ignore Proper Alignment*

Proper alignment is essential for a safe and productive practice. To obtain a deeper stretch, avoid ignoring alignment cues or sacrificing posture. Alignment is important because it assures safety, reduces accidents, and maximizes the benefits of each position.

8.   *Avoid Ignoring Pain or Discomfort:*

While some discomfort or minor stretching sensations are typical, severe pain or extreme discomfort are indicators of a problem. During practicing, avoid disregarding discomfort sensations. To avoid damage, alter the position or ease off if a movement creates intense pain or discomfort.

9. *Don't Forget About Mindfulness and Presence*

During your Chair Yoga practices, try not to let your thoughts wander or become distracted. Cultivate mindfulness and presence by paying attention to your body's sensations, your breath, and the present moment. Participating actively in the practice increases its efficacy.

10.   Do not skip warm-ups and cool-downs. Warm-ups prepare your body for practice, while cool-downs allow it to return to rest. Skip these important stages of your Chair Yoga session. Warm-ups prevent injuries, while cool-downs encourage relaxation and practice integration.

How to Creating a Comfortable Chair Yoga Space at Home:

Welcome to your personal retreat, a place where the embrace of serenity meets the flow of Chair Yoga practice. We'll go over step-by-step tactics and creative ideas for creating a comfortable, inviting, and conducive Chair Yoga room in the comfort of your own home in this complete guide. Let us go on this transformational and health journey together.

1. Choosing the Best Location

Considerations:

- Accessibility: Select a location with ample space for your chair and free movement.
- Natural Light: If feasible, choose a location with natural light to help create a relaxing atmosphere.
- Choose a quiet location to limit distractions and encourage attention during practice.
- Comfort: For a comfortable practice, make sure the location has a suitable temperature and adequate ventilation.

2. Laying the Groundwork

Elements of Transformation:

- Invest in a strong, comfortable chair that supports your posture and allows for simple mobility.
- Chair Positioning: Place the chair on a flat, even surface to provide stability and a clean area around it.

- Yoga Mat or Rug: To establish a specific practice space and offer padding for your feet, place a yoga mat or a soft rug beneath your chair.
- Comfortable Attire: Wear loose, breathable clothes that allows for unfettered mobility throughout practice.

3. Adding Ambience

Tranquility Elements:

- Ambient Lighting: To create a peaceful ambiance, use soft, soothing lighting such as lamps, candles, or dimmable lights.
- Aromatherapy: For relaxation and focus, consider diffusing essential oils such as lavender or eucalyptus
- Soft Music or Sounds: To improve the environment and help in relaxing, play soothing, instrumental music or natural sounds.

4. Individualization and Inspiration

Adding Your Touch:

- Personal additions like as artwork, plants, or furnishings that inspire and elevate your practice environment can be included as decorative elements.
- Motivating phrases or Affirmations: Display motivating phrases or affirmations that are relevant to your Chair Yoga adventure.
- Create a vision board or an inspiration zone with photos that represent your wellness objectives and dreams.

5. Organizational Considerations

Comfort and order:

- Yoga props and accessories should be carefully organized in baskets, shelves, or storage boxes for quick access.
- Decluttering: Keep the area neat and clutter-free during practice to encourage a sense of serenity and focus.

- Tech-Free Zone: Keep technological gadgets and distractions to a minimum in the environment to promote mindfulness and focus.

6. Rituals and mindfulness

Increasing Practice Time:

- Mindful Preparation: Set aside a few minutes before practice for breathing exercises, grounding, or intention setting.
- Make Good Use of Props: Yoga props such as blocks, belts, or cushions should be kept handy for support during postures.
- Guided Meditation or Closing Rituals: For a more comprehensive experience, incorporate brief meditation or gratitude rituals at the end of your sessions.

7. Consistency and Upkeep

Creating Sacred Spaces:

- Regular Cleaning and Maintenance: Keep your area clean and orderly to keep its holiness.

- Commit to frequent Chair Yoga practices in your designated location, establishing a sense of familiarity and ease.

8. Adaptability and flexibility

Accept Evolving Needs:

- Adaptability of environment: Be willing to rearrange or change things in your environment based on changing preferences or needs.
- Allow your area to change with your practice, incorporating new items that inspire and support your wellness journey.

9. Including Natural Elements

Bringing Nature Inside:

- Indoor Plants: Use potted plants or a small indoor garden to bring nature's calming impact into your room. To improve air quality, use plants recognized for their air-purifying properties.
- Natural Materials: To create an earthy and grounded mood, use décor or furniture made of

natural materials such as wood, bamboo, or eco-friendly textiles.

10. Simple Storage Options

Organizational Accessibility:

- Use open shelving, baskets, or wall-mounted organizers near your practice area for easy access. To eliminate disruptions during sessions, make sure yoga tools, towels, or water are easily accessible.
- Multipurpose Furniture: Look for items that act as storage containers to save space while keeping yoga basics close at hand.

14: Adaptable Mood Lighting:

Atmosphere Change:

- Install dimmer switches or utilize adjustable bulbs to change the lighting intensity and create different atmospheres appropriate for leisure or concentrate.

- colorful Lighting: During practice sessions, experiment with colorful light bulbs or LED strips to create atmosphere or foster various emotions.

Chapter 3: Breath and Body Warm-ups:

The Benefits of Chair Yoga Breathing Exercises

The art of attentive breathing intertwines with the fluidity of movement in the calm expanse of Chair Yoga, proclaiming a gateway to profound relaxation, heightened awareness, and total well-being. In this chapter, we'll look at the important advantages of chair yoga breathing exercises, including how they may improve physical health, mental clarity, and inner peace.

The Importance of Chair Yoga Breathing Exercises

Chair Yoga stresses the skill of mindful breathing, known as Pranayama in traditional yoga practice, as well as physical postures. These breathing exercises seek to harness the power of the breath, developing a stronger bond between body, mind, and spirit. You sit comfortably in your chair and begin a journey of controlled, purposeful breathwork, which unlocks a plethora of advantages.

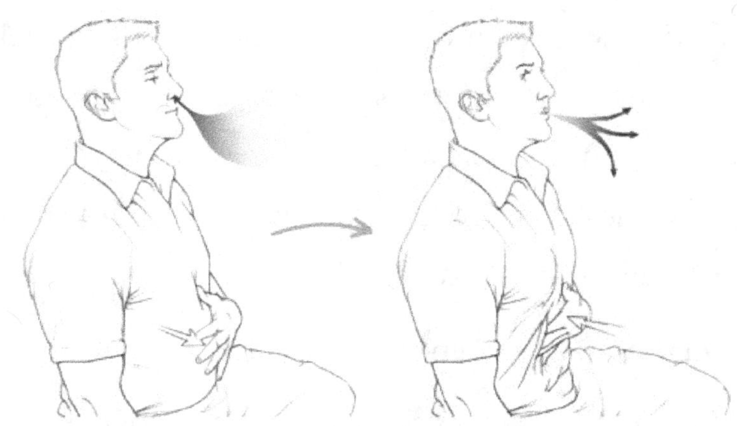

Breathing Exercises

1. Improving Respiratory Health

Description: Chair yoga breathing exercises are essential for improving respiratory functioning. Deep, diaphragmatic breaths increase lung capacity, enhancing oxygen intake and air circulation. As a result, respiratory muscles are strengthened, shallow breathing patterns are alleviated, and total lung efficiency is improved.

2. Relaxation and Stress Reduction

Description: Chair yoga breathing techniques are an effective stress and tension reliever. Slow, deliberate breathing patterns engage the parasympathetic nervous system, causing relaxation and tranquility. The practice calms the mind, decreases anxiety, and aids in the treatment of stress-related illnesses.

3. Increased Mindfulness and Clarity

Description: Chair yoga's deliberate concentration on breath cultivates awareness and mental clarity. The mind becomes more aware when attention is drawn to the regular flow of inhalations and exhalations. This improves focus, sharpens cognitive functioning, and increases mental clarity.

4. Emotional and Energy Balance

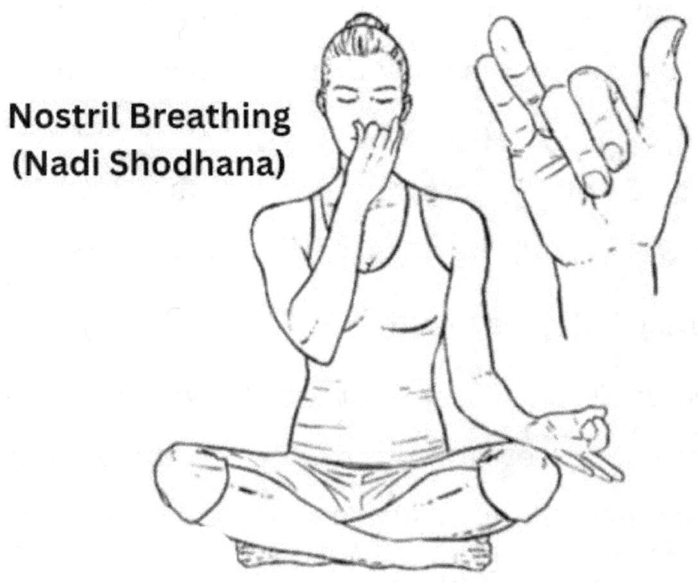

Description: Chair yoga breathing exercises promote emotional balance by regulating energy flow in the body. Techniques like as alternating nostril breathing (Nadi Shodhana) help to balance and stabilize the body's energy pathways. This helps with mood fluctuations and promotes a sense of well-being.

5. Increasing Body Awareness and Posture

Description: Chair yoga promotes greater posture and body awareness via mindful breathing. Individuals automatically align their spine and engage core muscles when they focus on deep, controlled breaths. This promotes healthy posture and spinal health by cultivating a heightened sense of body awareness.

6. Improving Digestive Health

Description: Certain chair yoga breathing methods, such as diaphragmatic breathing or belly breathing, activate the vagus nerve, increasing relaxation and assisting digestion. These methods improve digestion by minimizing bloating and increasing food absorption.

7. Immune Function Enhancement

Description: Regular chair yoga breathing exercises help to improve immune function. Deep breathing increases oxygenation, which strengthens the body's immunological response and its capacity to fight infections and diseases.

8. Pain and Discomfort Management

Description: Chair Yoga uses mindful breathing as a coping method to manage pain and discomfort. The practice instills a sense of serenity, lowering pain perception and cultivating a relaxed state in the midst of distress.

9. Combining Breath and Movement

Description: Chair yoga breathing techniques blend effortlessly with movement to create a coordinated flow. Coordination of breath and moderate movements increases the advantages, deepening stretches and improving relaxation.

Chair Yoga Gentle Warm-ups and Stretches: Nurturing Body and Mind

The trip begins in the peaceful embrace of Chair Yoga with moderate yet vigorous warm-up movements and stretches meant to awaken the body, enhance flexibility, and set the way for a harmonious practice. This chapter digs into a number of customized exercises, investigating their advantages, methodologies, and the transforming potential they bring to your Chair Yoga sessions.

1. Seated Neck Stretches

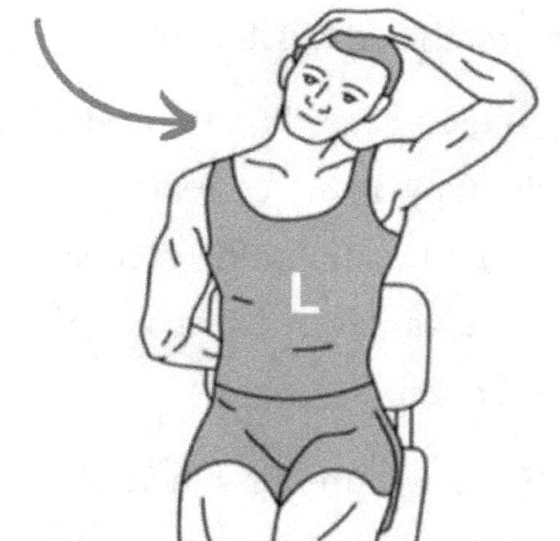

Seated Neck Stretches Yoga

Seated neck stretches in Chair Yoga relieve stress and stiffness. To deepen the stretch, tilt your head to the right and gently pull it with your right hand. Hold for a few breaths and then switch sides. This exercise promotes relaxation by increasing neck mobility and decreasing neck tension.

2. Shoulder Releases and Rolls

Lift your shoulders up, roll them backward, and then down in a circular motion to perform shoulder rolls. This exercise relaxes the shoulders, increases circulation, and promotes a relaxed posture.

3. Spinal Twists

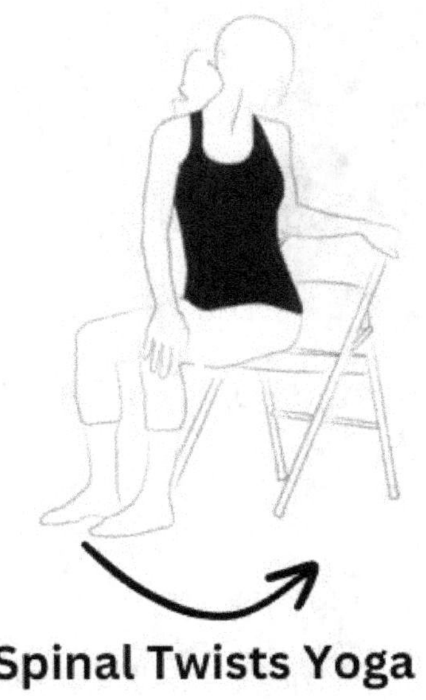

Spinal Twists Yoga

Seated spinal twists entail gradually twisting the upper body to either side while supported by the chair's back or armrest. This exercise relieves back strain, improves flexibility, and promotes digestion.

4. Seated Forward Fold

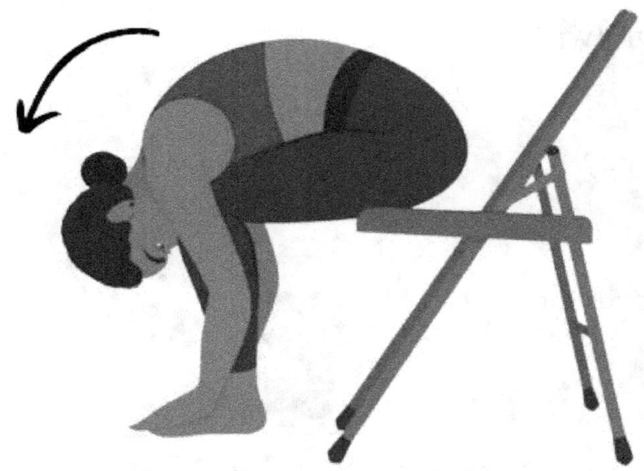

Seated Forward Fold Yoga

Seated forward folds stretch the back, hamstrings, and hip flexors. Sit on the chair's edge, tilt forward from your hips, and reach for your toes or the floor. This stretch increases hamstring flexibility while also relaxing the lower back.

5. Gentle Leg Extensions

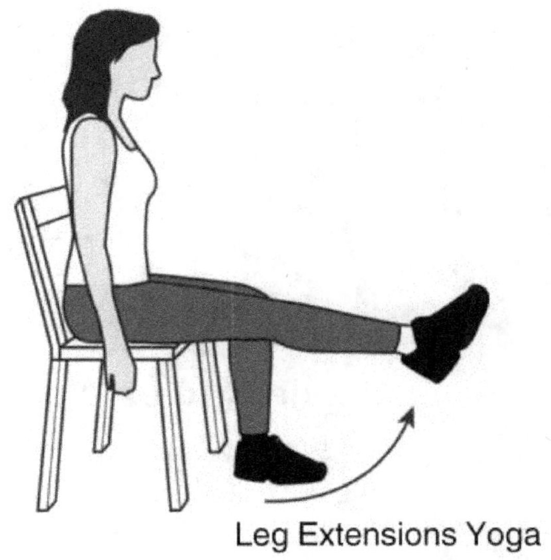

Leg Extensions Yoga

Extend one leg forward with the foot flexed, hold for a few seconds, and then lower it. Alter between the legs.

This exercise strengthens the legs, stretches the hamstrings, and improves circulation in the lower body.

5. Circles around the ankles

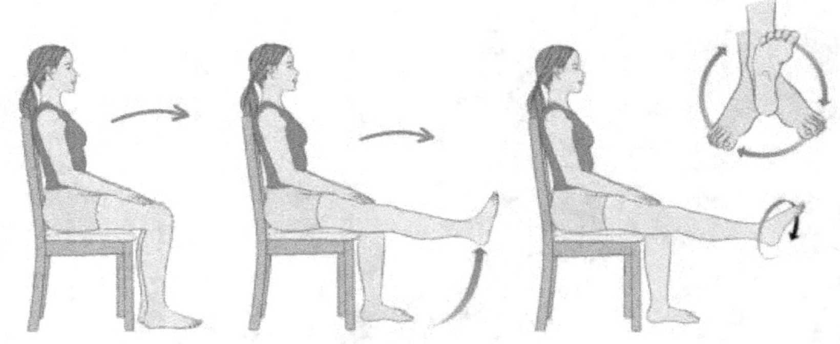

Ankle Circles Yoga

Lift one foot off the ground and spin your ankle in a circular manner. Reverse the process in both clockwise and counterclockwise directions. Ankle circles promote ankle flexibility, ankle strength, and circulation in the foot.

6. Seated Chest Opener.

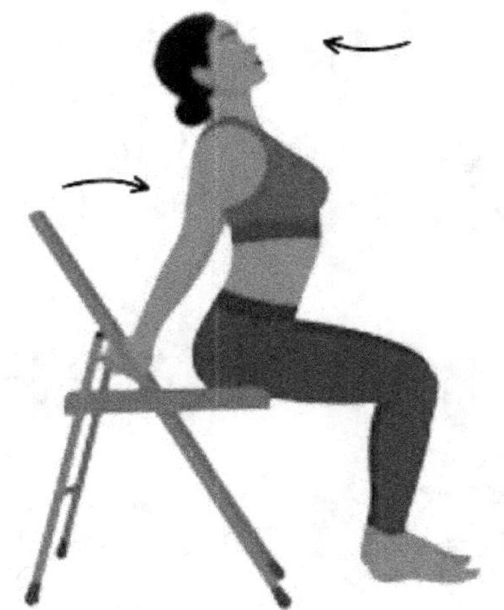

Seated Chest Opener Yoga

Sit on the chair's edge, interlace your fingers behind your back, and gradually elevate your arms while opening your chest. This stretch helps to correct rounded shoulders, enhance posture, and open the chest.

7. Seated Cat-Cow Stretch

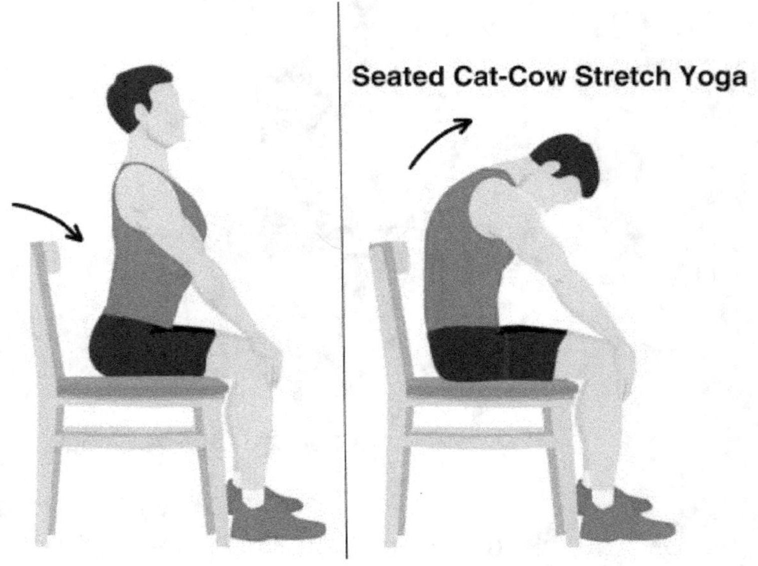

Sit up straight in your chair, lay your hands on your thighs, and alternate arching (cow) and rounding (cat) your back. This stretch relieves spinal stress, soothes the back muscles, and increases spinal flexibility.

Key Points from Breathing and Warm-up routines.

Breathing Exercises:

- ✓ Prioritize breath quality above quantity, concentrating on calm, deep inhalations and exhalations.
- ✓ Engage in conscious breathing throughout warm-ups, synchronizing breath with movement for a harmonic practice.
- ✓ To increase lung capacity and induce calm, practice diaphragmatic breathing.
- ✓ Instead of holding your breath, maintain a constant and regular flow of breath throughout the exercises.
- ✓ Beyond the practice, embrace breath awareness by incorporating mindful breathing into everyday activities for general well-being.

Warm-Up Stretches:

✓ Warm up your muscles and prepare your body for movement by starting your Chair Yoga practice with simple stretches.

✓ Maintain a comfortable and pain-free range of motion during stretches by focusing on good alignment.

✓ Respect your body's limitations and prevent overexertion by moving gently and thoughtfully into each stretch.

✓ Pay attention to your body's cues; if a stretch produces discomfort or agony, back off or change your posture.

✓ Warm-up stretches should be done on a regular basis to increase flexibility, circulation, and relieve stress in the body.

Patience and consistency:

✓ Make a habit of adding breathing exercises and warm-ups into your everyday Chair Yoga practice.

✓ be patient and gentle with yourself. Allow for steady growth in flexibility and breath awareness.

✓ Respect your body's rate of improvement by avoiding harsh activities and expecting results right away.

✓ Accept the road of self-discovery and progress by practicing consistently and engaging mindfully.

✓ Celebrate small achievements and improvement in breath control, flexibility, and overall well-being.

Chapter 4, 25-Day Chair Yoga journey (Beginner Level)

Begin a transforming 25-day Chair Yoga journey designed for beginners who want to improve their posture and experience the uplifting effects of mindful movement. These easy yet powerful postures have been painstakingly crafted to progressively strengthen the spine, increase alignment, and foster a more upright, balanced posture. Let's take this inspiring journey together, one posture at a time.

Week 1: Laying the Groundwork

1. Seated Mountain Pose (Tadasana Variation)
    - Sit tall on your chair, with both feet on the ground, ankles beneath knees, and hips stacked over ankles.
    - Extend the arms alongside the body, lengthen the spine, activate core muscles, and relax shoulders.

- Visualize yourself as a mountain, cultivating awareness of spinal alignment and core activation.

2. Seated Cat-Cow Stretch:

   - Sit forward in your chair, hands on your thighs, and arch your back on inhalation (Cow) and round it on exhale (Cat).
   - Breathe in and out, gradually mobilizing the spine and increasing spinal flexibility.

Week 2: Welcome Back Strength

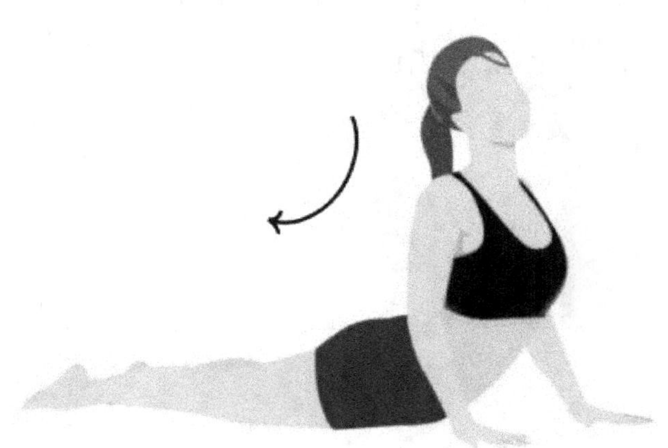

Cobra Pose Yoga

1. Seated Backbend:

- Sit on the chair's edge, placing your hands on your lower back for support, and gradually lean back, elevating your chest.
- Engage your abdominal muscles to cushion your lower back, expand your chest, and prevent hunching.

2. Cobra Pose:

- Sit forward on the chair, lay your hands on the seat's edge, and gradually elevate your chest to lengthen your spine.
- Concentrate on lengthening the front body, stretching the belly, and expanding the area around the heart.

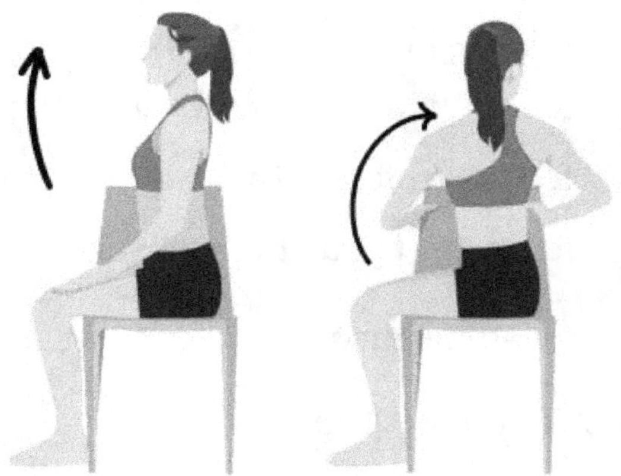

Mild Seated Twist

1. Seated Spinal Twist:

   - Sit tall, inhale to stretch the spine, and exhale to gently twist to one side, utilizing the back of the chair for support.

   - Maintain spine length, deepen the twist with each exhale, and then repeat on the opposite side.

2. Eagle Arms Stretch:

- Cross one arm beneath the other, bend your elbows, and bring your hands together or touch opposing shoulders.
- Raise your elbows to shoulder height and feel a stretch between your shoulder blades to expand your upper back.

Week 4: Improved Balance and Alignment

1. Half-Moon Pose (Seated):
    - Sit on the chair's edge, lay one hand on the seat, and extend the opposing arm above to create a side stretch.
    - Engage the core muscles, lengthen the spine, and slowly lean to the side to feel a stretch down the torso.
2. Chair Supported Warrior Pose:
    - Sit forward on the chair, one foot back, one foot forward, and arms aloft, facing forward.
    - Root down into the sitting bones, engage the core, and feel the spine's strength and length.

Chair Yoga Poses to Improve Mobility for Beginners

Welcome to Chair Yoga's portal to movement and release. This chapter is a carefully crafted journey of moderate yet effective postures for beginners looking to increase mobility, flexibility, and total body functionality. Each position is designed to energize joints, lengthen muscles, and increase range of motion, allowing beginners to appreciate the transformational effects of mindful movement.

Week 1: Joint Awakening

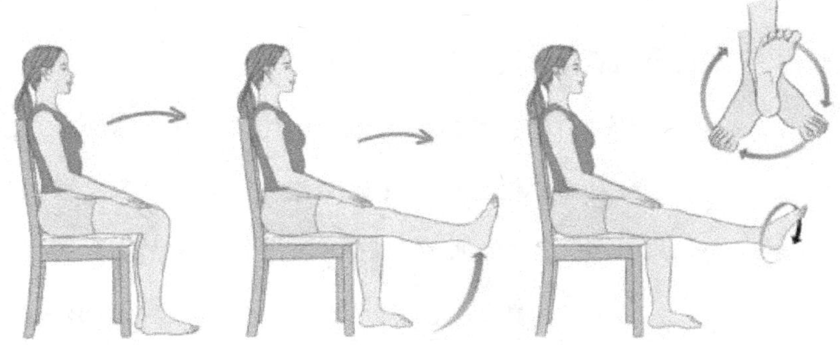

Ankle Circles Yoga

1. Ankles Circles:

    - Sit up straight, raise one foot, and spin the ankle in a circular motion.

    - Rotate the ankles clockwise and counterclockwise to move the joints and increase circulation in the feet.

2. Wrist Rotations:

    - Extend your arms to shoulder height and spin your wrists clockwise and counterclockwise.

    - This exercise improves wrist flexibility and strength, which is useful for everyday tasks and hand mobility.

Week 2 focuses on hip and knee flexibility.

1. Seated Knee-to-Chest Stretch:

    - Sit up straight and hug one knee to the chest with both hands.

    - Feel the stretch in your hips and lower back as you alternate legs to improve hip flexibility.

2. Seated Leg Extensions,

- Sit on the chair's edge and stretch one leg forward, keeping the foot flexible.
- Alternate legs, feeling the hamstring stretch and improving knee mobility.

Week 3: Increase Your Spinal Flexibility

1. Twist when seated:

- Sit tall, inhale to stretch the spine, and exhale to twist slightly to one side.
- Use the chair's back for support, allowing you to feel the stretch along your spine and improve spinal mobility.

2. Forward Fold Chair Supported:

- Sit forward in your chair, hinge at the hips, and softly fold forward, aiming for your shins or the floor.
- Feel the stretch throughout your spine and hamstrings, which will improve spinal flexibility and relieve stress.

Week 4: Mobility of the Shoulders and Upper Body

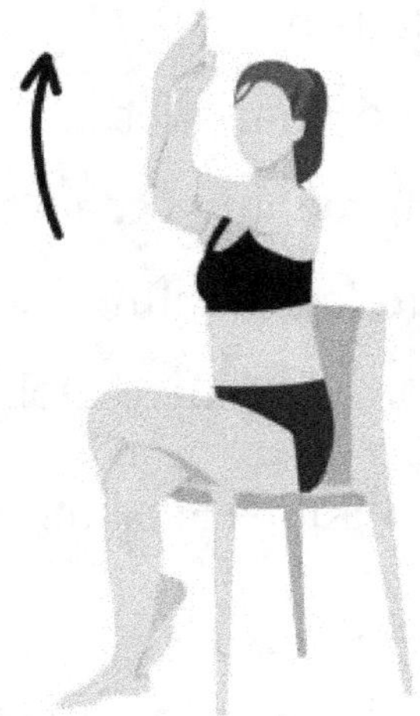

Eagle Arms Stretch

1. Shoulders Rolls:

   - Sit tall and exhale to rotate your shoulders backward and downward.

   - To relieve stress and enhance shoulder mobility, perform slow and controlled shoulder rolls.

2. Eagle Arms Stretch:

   - Cross one arm over the other, bend your elbows, and bring your hands together or contact your shoulders.

- To improve upper body mobility, raise your elbows to shoulder height and feel a stretch between your shoulder blades.

Chair Yoga Poses for Cardiovascular Health and Stamina Building

Welcome to a journey focusing on heart health and stamina building via attentive Chair Yoga practices. These exercises have been carefully selected for beginners with the goal of improving heart health, increasing endurance, and cultivating energy. Accept these simple yet empowering stances to progressively energize the cardiovascular system and improve stamina.

Week 1: Increasing Circulation

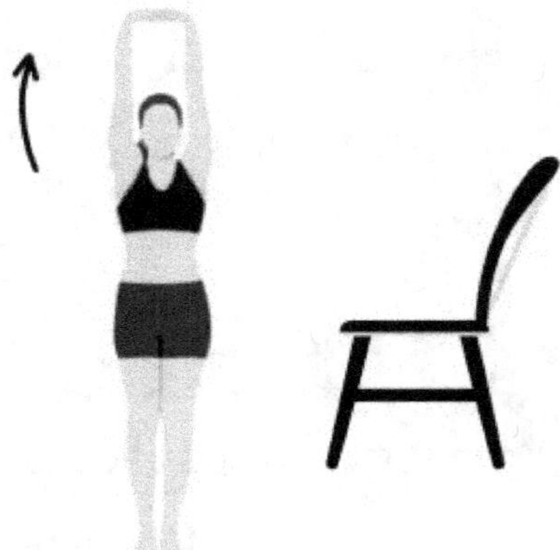

Mountain Pose Tadasana

1. Seated Mountain Pose (Tadasana Variation),

    - Sit tall, with both feet on the ground, ankles beneath knees, and hips stacked over ankles.

    - Extend your arms alongside your body, palms facing inward, to increase circulation and grounding.

2. Seated Forward Fold:

    - Sit on the chair's edge and tilt forward from the hips, aiming toward the floor or shins.

- Improves blood circulation, extends the spine, and promotes relaxation, all of which benefit heart health.

Week 2: Activating the Core

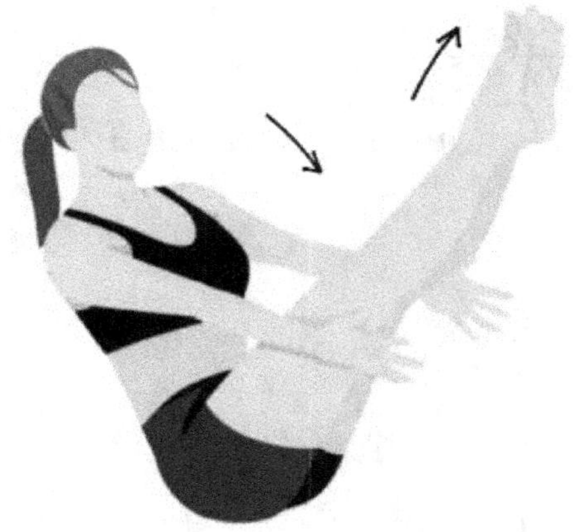

Boat Pose Yoga

1. Chair-Supported Warrior Pose:
   - Sit in the chair, one foot back, and lift your arms high, staring forward.

- Engages core muscles, strengthens legs, and increases circulation, all of which benefit heart health.

2. Seated Boat Pose Variation:

   - Sit forward, elevate your legs, then lean back slightly to form a "V" shape with your body.
   - Engages core muscles, increasing strength and endurance and benefiting heart health.

Week 3: Energizing the Body,

1. Seated Spinal Twist:

   - Sit tall, inhale to stretch the spine, and exhale to gently twist to one side, supported by the chair's back.
   - Circulation is increased, abdominal organs are massaged, and the heart is stimulated.

2. Camel Pose with a Chair:

- Sit tall, grip the chair's sides, arch your back, and elevate your chest, staring skyward.
- Stretches the front of the body, energizes the spine, and improves heart health.

Week 4: Elevation Via Breath

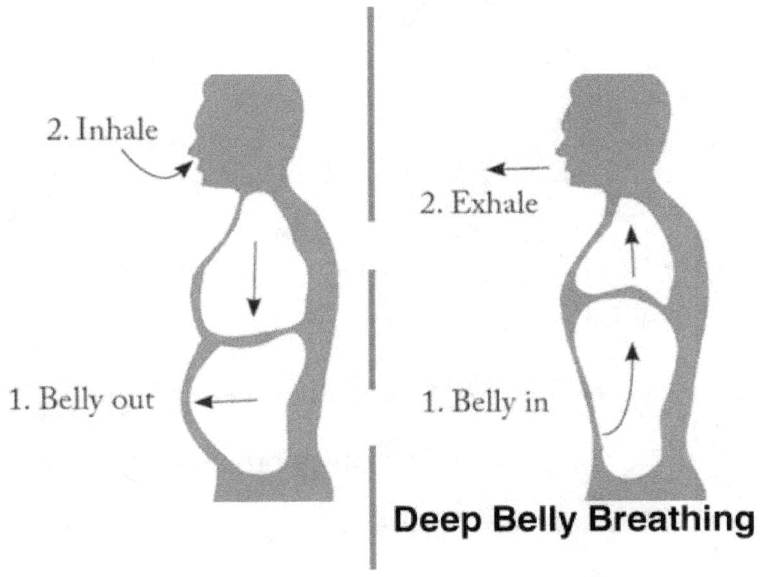

1. Diaphragmatic Breathing (Deep Belly Breathing):
   - Place one hand on the tummy and one hand on the chest and sit comfortably.

- Deeply inhale through the nose, extending the abdomen, and slowly exhale through the mouth.
- By soothing the nervous system, it improves oxygenation, calms the body, and promotes heart health.

2. Deep Breathing in the Mountain Pose:

- Sit tall, breathe deeply, and lift your arms aloft. Exhale gently while lowering your arms.
- Combines breath and movement to promote calm and heart-centered awareness.

Chair Yoga Poses for Weight Loss

Welcome to a transforming journey in which Chair Yoga becomes a weight loss buddy. These beginner-friendly poses are designed to stimulate metabolism, improve circulation, and increase body awareness, supporting a slow but effective approach to weight loss. Accept these gentle motions to help you lose weight while also soothing your body and mind.

Week 1: Igniting Metabolism,

1. Seated Cat-Cow Stretch:

    - Sit forward in your chair, hands on your thighs, and arch your back on inhalation (Cow) and round it on exhale (Cat).
    - Stimulates the spine, activates core muscles, and revs up metabolism.

2. Seated Forward Fold:

    - Sit on the chair's edge and tilt forward from the hips, aiming toward the floor or shins.
    - Activates abdominal muscles, stretches the back, and helps digestion, all of which contribute to weight loss.

Week 2: Activating the Core Muscles

1. Seated Knee-to-Chest Stretch:

    - Sit up straight and hug one knee to the chest with both hands.
    - It works the stomach muscles, massages the internal organs, and aids digestion.

2. Chair-Supported Boat Pose Variation:

- Sit forward, elevate your legs, and lean back slightly, forming a "V" shape with your body while grasping the chair's sides.
- Engages core muscles, strengthens abdominal muscles, and assists in midsection toning.

Week 3: Improving Circulation

1. Seated Twist:
   - Sit tall, inhale to stretch the spine, and exhale to gently twist to one side, supported by the chair's back.
   - It stimulates digestion, increases circulation, and aids in detoxifying.
2. Stretch Seated Side Bend:
   - Sit tall, extend one arm above, and slowly lean to the other side, feeling the torso expand.
   - Stretches the sides, increases flexibility, and aids lymph drainage.

Week 4: Movement and Mindful Breathing

1. Diaphragmatic Breathing (Deep Belly Breathing):

   - Place one hand on the tummy and one hand on the chest and sit comfortably.

   - Deeply inhale through the nose, extending the abdomen, and slowly exhale through the mouth.

   - Relaxes the body, decreases stress-related eating, and encourages mindful eating practices.

2. Mountain Pose with Deep Breathing:

   - Sit tall, breathe deeply, lift your arms high, and exhale gently while lowering your arms.

   - Integrates breath with movement, developing awareness and assisting in stress management, which can have a favorable influence on weight reduction.

25-Day Chair Yoga Challenge for Beginners

Welcome to a life-changing 25-day Chair Yoga program tailored exclusively for beginners. This challenge is designed to gradually and easily introduce basic postures, breathing exercises, and mindful practices. Follow this step-by-step tutorial to get the advantages of Chair Yoga, which promotes physical and mental well-being.

Day 1-5: Laying the Groundwork

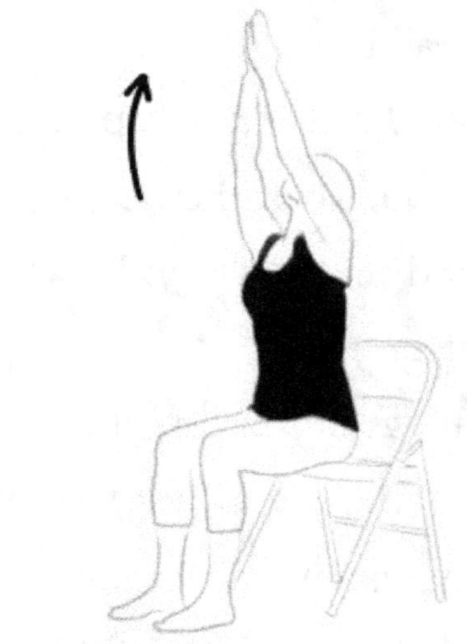

Mountain Posture Yoga

Day 1: Seated Mountain Pose (Tadasana Variation)

- Sit tall on a chair, with both feet on the ground, ankles beneath knees, and hips stacked over ankles.
- Extend your arms beside your body, palms facing in, to promote stability and grounding.

Day 2: Seated Cat-Cow Stretch,

- it forward in your chair, hands on your thighs, and arch your back on inhalation (Cow) and round it on exhale (Cat).
- Gently move the spine, activating core muscles and increasing flexibility.

Day 3 Seated Knee-to-Chest Stretch,

- Sit tall and hug one knee to the chest with both hands, feeling the stretch in your hips and lower back.
- Improve hip flexibility and relieve lower-body stress.

Day 4: Seated Forward Fold,

- Sit on the chair's edge and tilt forward from the hips, aiming toward the floor or shins.
- A mild forward fold stretches the spine and hamstrings while also promoting calm.

Day 5: Diaphragmatic Breathing (Deep Belly Breathing)

- Place one hand on the tummy and one hand on the chest and sit comfortably.
- Deeply inhale via the nose, expanding the belly, and slowly exhale through the mouth, promoting calm and attention.

Day 6–10: Accepting Flexibility

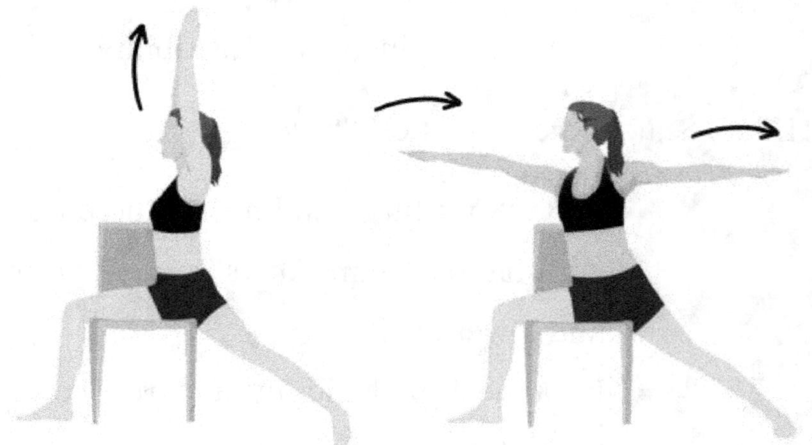

Warrior Pose Yoga

Day 6: Seated Spinal Twist,

- Sit tall, inhale to stretch the spine, and exhale to gently twist to one side, supported by the chair's back.
- Gentle twists improve spinal flexibility and increase digestion.

Day 7: Seated Leg Extensions,

- Sit on the chair's edge and stretch one leg forward, keeping the foot flexible.
- Enhance hamstring flexibility and circulation in the legs.

Day 8: Chair Supported Warrior Pose:

- Sit forward in your chair, take one foot back, and raise your arms above, using your core muscles and increasing your strength.

Day 9: Seated Boat Pose Variation:

- Sit up straight, elevate your legs, and lean back slightly, working your core muscles to strengthen your abdomen and enhance your balance.

Day 10: Chair Supported Backbend:

- Sit on the chair's edge, rest your hands on your lower back for support, softly lean back, and elevate your chest.
- Open the front of the body, improve back flexibility, and activate the heart center.

Day 11-15: Mindfulness Practice

Day 11: Mountain Pose with Deep Breathing:

- Sit tall, inhale deeply, and lift your arms aloft. Exhale slowly while lowering your arms, blending breath and movement.

Day 12: Seated Forward Fold with Chair Support:

- Sit forward in your chair, hinge at the hips, and softly fold forward, aiming for your shins or the floor.
- A supported forward fold can help you relax and improve your flexibility.

Day 13: Seated Eagle Arms Stretch

- Cross one arm over the other, bend your elbows, and bring your hands together or contact your shoulders.
- Improve mobility and posture by releasing tension in the upper back and shoulders.

Day 14: Seated Side Bend Stretch

- Sit tall, extend one arm above, and slowly lean to the other side, feeling the torso expand.
- Increase lateral flexibility and respiratory capacity.

Day 15: Mindful Body Scan Meditation

- Close your eyes and bring your focus to different regions of your body, noticing feelings without judgment.
- A guided body scan meditation can help you become more self-aware and relax.

Day 16-20: Strengthening

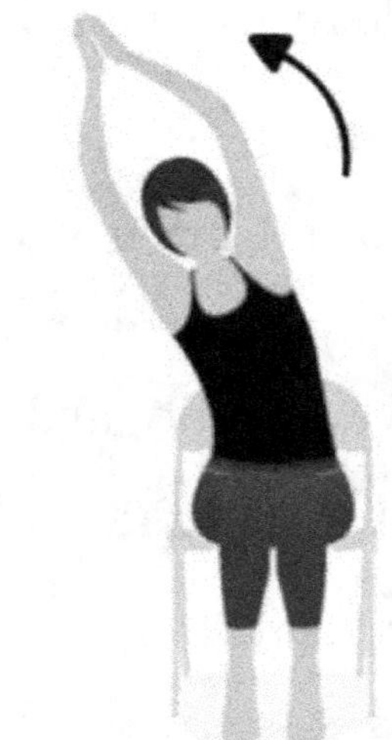

Crescent Moon Stretch

Day 16: Seated Warrior Pose

- To promote strength and stability, sit tall, extend one leg back, activate core muscles, and reach arms aloft.

Day 17: Seated Crescent Moon Stretch

- Sit tall, interlace your fingers and raise your arms aloft, then slowly lean to one side to feel a stretch throughout your torso.

- Increase side body flexibility and circulation.

Day 18: Seated Chest Opener

- Sit on the chair, interlace your fingers behind your back, and gradually lift your arms to open your chest and shoulders.
- Reduce slouching, improve posture, and increase breathing capacity.

Day 19: Seated Twist with Eagle Arms Variation

- Sit up straight, cross one arm under the other, bend your elbows, and slowly twist, working core muscles and increasing spinal flexibility.

Day 20: Forward Fold Twist with Chair Support

- Sit forward in the chair, twist to one side, support yourself by holding the chair's back, and fold forward gently.
- A slight twist and forward fold can improve spinal mobility and accelerate digestion.

Day 21-25: Flow and Integration

Day 21: Seated Flow Sequence

- Combine acquired positions in a seamless sequence, going from one pose to the next while breathing mindfully.

Day 22: Seated Balance Poses

Lifting one foot, using core muscles, and establishing stability are all examples of easy balance poses.

Day 23: Mantra Seated Meditation

- Close your eyes and softly recite a relaxing mantra or affirmation to promote attention and inner tranquility.

Day 24: Chair Yoga Mindfulness Walk

- Take a brief, thoughtful stroll, paying attention to each stride, posture, and breath, combining movement with mindfulness.

Day 25: Flow of Celebration

- Revisit favorite challenging poses while moving through a flow sequence, applauding progress, and practicing mindfulness.

key points to remember as a beginner in Chair Yoga:

✓ Begin slowly: Begin with easy positions and work your way up to more complicated ones as your body adjusts.

✓ Pay Attention to Your Body: Respect your body's limitations and never push a position. If something is difficult or painful, take it slowly.

✓ Concentrate on Breathing: Breathing is essential. To enhance your practice and stay present, connect your motions with your breath.

✓ Use Props for Support: Chairs, pillows, and blocks may be great for stability and support while you experiment with positions.

- ✓ Maintain Good Posture: Sit up straight and activate your core. Good posture ensures that practice is both safe and effective.

- ✓ Consistency trumps intensity: Practice on a regular basis, even if just for a few minutes. Pushing too hard in a single session is less crucial than consistency.

- ✓ Patience is essential: It takes time to see results. Be kind with yourself and enjoy the ride without hurrying.

- ✓ Modify as Needed: Feel free to change the positions to suit your comfort level or to accommodate any physical constraints.

- ✓ Keep water close by and hydrate yourself before, during, and after your practice.

- ✓ Warm-up and cool-down: Always warm up before attempting positions, and include a cool-down session at the end to calm your body and mind.

✓ Seek Advice: If at all feasible, try enrolling in a beginner's class or following reputable tutorials to guarantee appropriate form and technique.

✓ Take Advantage of the Opportunity: Accept Chair Yoga as a comprehensive practice that not only improves the body but also the mind and spirit.

Chapter 5: Chair Yoga Journey (Intermediate Level) for 25 Days

Welcome to an energizing 25-day Chair Yoga experience designed for people progressing from beginning to advanced levels. This program is intended to improve posture, mobility, heart health, and weight control. Accept these intermediate-level positions and practices to strengthen your relationship with your body and mind.

Day 1–5: Posture Improvement

Suggestion for an image: A person seated on a chair displaying an improved seated mountain position.

Day 1: Refinement of Seated Mountain Pose (Tadasana Variation)

- Improve your sitting mountain pose by focusing on grounding, engaging core muscles, and elongating the spine.

Day 2: Refinement of the Seated Forward Fold

- Deepen the sitting forward fold by emphasizing spine lengthening and stretching towards the floor or shins.

Day 3: Variation of the Seated Cat-Cow Stretch

- Experiment with several cat-cow stretches, increasing spinal flexion and extension while syncing breath.

Day 4: Progression of Seated Backbends

- Increase the difficulty of sitting backbends by activating core muscles, expanding the chest, and deepening the stretch.

Day 5: Seated Twist Progression

- Introduce advanced sitting twists, deepen the rotation, and use breath to explore spinal mobility further.

Day 6–10: Mobility Improvement

Day 6: Variation of the Knee-to-Chest Stretch

- Deeper knee-to-chest stretches, activating hip flexors, and stretching the lower back are all options.

Day 7: Refinement of Seated Leg Extensions

- Maintain appropriate posture while progressing in sitting leg extensions and deepening the strain in the hamstrings.

Day 8: Refinement of the Chair Supported Warrior Pose

- Advance chair-supported warrior postures while exercising core muscles and maintaining balance and stability.

Day 9: Progression of the Seated Boat Pose

- Deepen sitting boat pose variations by strengthening the core and achieving balance in difficult positions.

Day 10: Progression of the Chair Supported Camel Pose

- Advance in chair-supported camel postures, opening the front body, and increasing spinal flexibility.

Day 11-15: Cardiovascular Health and Stamina

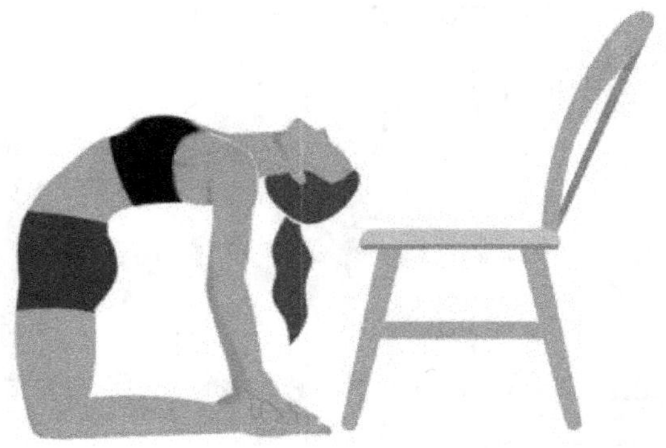

Camel Pose Yoga

Day 11: Heart-Opening Poses on a Chair

- Concentrate on heart-opening positions with chair support to promote emotional release and circulation.

Day 12: Variation of the Seated Side Bend Stretch

- Deeper sitting side bend stretches can improve lateral flexibility and encourage deeper breathing.

Day 13: Forward Bend Twist with Chair Support

- Make progress with chair-supported forward bend twists, which stimulate digestion and promote spinal health.

Day 14: Seated Warrior Pose Series

- Sequence sitting warrior postures to build lower-body strength, stability, and endurance.

Day 15: Variation of Chair Supported Standing Poses

- Introduce chair-supported standing postures to help improve balance and stamina.

Day 16-20: Poses for Weight Loss

Day 16: Core Strengthening with a Chair

- Concentrate on chair-supported core workouts, abdominal muscular engagement, and weight control.

Day 17: Seated Twist and Reach Progression

- Increase the difficulty of sitting twist and reach workouts by targeting the obliques and increasing spinal mobility.

Day 18: Leg Lifts Supported by a Chair

- Include chair-supported leg raises to help develop lower body muscles and promote stability.

Day 19: Series of Seated Balance Poses

- Sequence sitting balance poses to improve stability, attention, and weight-bearing capability.

Day 20: Chair-Supported High-Intensity Interval Training (HIIT)

- Introduce chair-supported HIIT activities for cardiovascular benefits, involving bursts of action and rest periods.

Days 21-25: Integration and Mastery

Day 21: Advanced Chair Yoga Flow Sequence

- In a flowing sequence, combine learned intermediate-level postures, integrating breath with movement.

Day 22: Chair-Supported Inversions and Extensions

- Investigate chair-supported inversions and extensions while progressively increasing strength and flexibility.

Day 23: Chair Supported Backbends Advanced

- Improve spinal flexibility and heart-opening feelings with chair-supported backbends.

Day 24: Forward Folds with Twists on a Chair

- Twist chair-supported forward folds to encourage cleansing and renewal.

Day 25: Flow of Mastery and Reflection

Create a flow sequence that incorporates mastered postures while also celebrating success and reflecting on the trip.

An Intermediate-Level Yoga Challenge for Consistent Improvement

Welcome to the Intermediate-Level Yoga Challenge, an energizing and transforming experience. This comprehensive program is designed to take your yoga practice to the next level by concentrating on increasing your flexibility, strength, mindfulness, and general well-being over a specified period of time. Accept these challenges to strengthen your connection with your mind, body, and soul.

Week 1: Focus on Flexibility

Day 1: Seated Twists Advanced

- Deepen sitting twists by experimenting with different arm placements and spinal rotations for increased flexibility.

Day 2: Longer Forward Folds

- In order to deepen the stretch in the hamstrings and spine, increase the intensity of forward folds by utilizing props or variants.

Day 3: Hip Opening Exercises with Progressions

- To enhance hip flexibility, begin with hip-opening exercises and progress to deeper stretches.

Day 4: Increased Side Bends

- Side bends should be progressed, with emphasis on elongation across the sides of the body for better lateral flexibility.

Day 5: Flow of Total Flexibility

- Combine learned flexibility postures into a flowing sequence, synchronizing breath and movement for a smooth flow.

Week 2: Strength Building

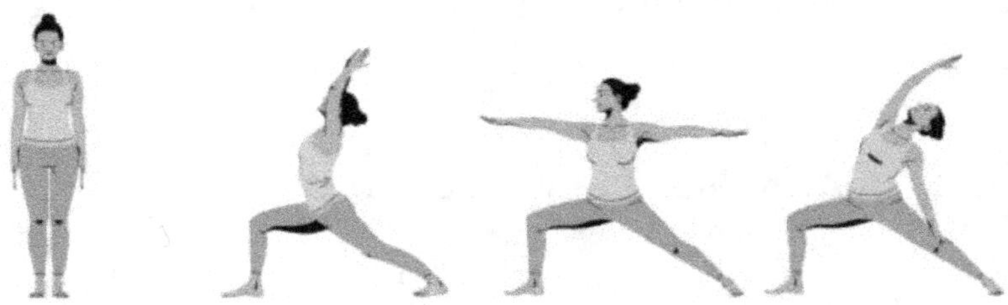

Warrior Stances Yoga

Day 6: Warrior Poses Supported by a Chair

- For strength, try warrior postures with a chair for support, targeting leg muscles and core stability.

Day 7: Core Strengthening Exercises

- Introduce rigorous core workouts that emphasize stomach and back muscular stability and strength.

Day 8: Chair-Assisted Inversions

- Working on upper body strength and balance, progress to inverted positions with chair support.

Day 9: Arm Balances with Changes

- Explore arm balancing postures with intermediate-level variants to improve strength and attention.

Day 10: Strength Fusion Flow

- Incorporate learned strength-building postures into a dynamic sequence to promote endurance and resilience.

Week 3: Balance and Mindfulness

Day 11: Advanced Meditation Techniques

- Investigate sophisticated meditation methods that use breathwork and imagery for increased awareness.

Day 12: Pranayama Mastery

- Devote a session to pranayama, or advanced breathing methods for increased consciousness.

Day 13: Balance Issues

- Introduce advanced balancing postures to help you improve your attention, stability, and proprioception.

Day 14: Sequencing Mindful Movements

- Create a mindful flow sequence that combines breath and movement for increased consciousness.

Day 15: Restorative and Yin Yoga

- Finish the week with restorative and yin yoga, which will allow the body to submit and relax fully.

Week 4: Whole-Body Integration

Day 16: Full Body Flow

- Participate in a full yoga sequence that incorporates components of flexibility, strength, awareness, and balance.

Day 17: Yoga Nidra Progressive

- Experiment with longer Yoga Nidra sessions to promote relaxation and subconscious investigation.

Day 18: Chakra Balancing Workshop

- Participate in a chakra-balancing session to harmonize energy centers for overall well-being.

Day 19: Partner Yoga Experiment

- Participate in partner yoga to strengthen your connection, trust, and communication with a partner or friend.

Day 20: Closing Ceremony and Reflection

- Finish the challenge with a closing ceremony that reflects on your progress, insights, and fresh views.

Navigating the 25-Day Intermediate-Level Yoga Challenge

Welcome to a life-changing 25-day yoga program designed for intermediate practitioners. This challenge intends to test limits, sharpen skills, and strengthen the bond between mind, body, and spirit. Every day presents a new chance for personal development and self-discovery.

Day 1-5: Expansion of Flexibility

Day 1: Seated Twists in Progress

- Begin with basic sitting twists and progressively increase the intensity by experimenting with variations and deeper rotations.

Day 2: Longer Forward Folds

- In forward folds, concentrate on stretching the spine and deepening the stretch with props or adjustments.

Day 3: Hip Opening Experiment

- Engage in hip-opening positions, progressively increasing the intensity of stretches to increase hip joint mobility.

Day 4: Focus on Lateral Flexibility

- Include side bends to lengthen the sides of the body and increase the range of motion in the torso.

Day 5: Flow of Harmonious Flexibility

- Integrate accomplished flexibility postures into a flowing sequence by coordinating breath with movement.

Day 6-10: Increased Strength and Stability

Day 6: Refinement of Chair-Supported Warrior Poses

- Increase the difficulty of the warrior poses by using a chair for stability and deeper participation.

Day 7: Core Strengthening Exercises

- For increased strength, concentrate on advanced core workouts that target deep abdominal and back muscles.

Day 8: Inversions with Chair Support

- Explore inverted postures with chair support, focusing on improving upper body strength and balance in inverted positions.

Day 9: Arm Balances and Change

- Explore arm balancing postures that may be modified to improve upper body strength and mental focus.

Day 10: Strength Fusion Flow

- In practice, incorporate taught strength-building postures into a dynamic flow to promote endurance and resilience.

Day 11-15: Increased Mindfulness and Balance

Day 11: Advanced Meditation Techniques

- Investigate deeper meditation methods that use pranayama and imagery for increased awareness.

Day 12: Pranayama Mastery

- Devote a session to pranayama methods and deeper breathwork for increased mindfulness.

Day 13: Advanced Balance Tests

- Practice sophisticated balance postures to improve your stability, attention, and proprioception.

Day 14: Sequencing Mindful Movements

- Create a sequence that delicately blends breath and movement, enhancing attention with each transition.

Day 15: Restorative and Yin Yoga Practice

- Finish the week with restorative and yin yoga, which promote deep relaxation and tissue release.

Day 16-20: Holistic Integration

Day 16: Complete Yoga Flow

- Engage in a lengthy yoga sequence that incorporates components of flexibility, strength, awareness, and balance.

Day 17: Yoga Nidra Session (Extended)

- Investigate prolonged Yoga Nidra, which encourages profound relaxation, subconscious investigation, and regeneration.

Day 18: Chakra Balancing Workshop

- Investigate chakra-balancing methods for harmonizing energy centers for overall well-being.

Day 19: Yoga with a Partner

- Practice partner yoga with a partner or a friend to build trust, connection, and mutual support.

Day 20: Closing Ceremony and Self-Reflection

- Finish the challenge with a closing ceremony that reflects on personal growth, insights, and accomplishments.

Day 21-25: Culmination and Mastery

Day 21: Progressive Yoga Flow

- Create a comprehensive yoga sequence by combining learned postures and transitions to enhance the flow experience.

Day 22: Relaxation and extended Yoga Nidra

- Dive further into Yoga Nidra for deep relaxation, renewal, and mental clarity.

Day 23: Advanced Pranayama Techniques

- Investigate complicated pranayama methods for improving breath control and creating awareness.

Day 24: Mastery of Inversions and Play

- Concentrate on mastering inversions without the use of props, stressing good alignment and developing confidence in inverted positions.

Day 25: Self-Evaluation and Celebration

- Celebrate the challenge's completion with a personal celebration and reflection session. Evaluate your journey's progress, insights, and fresh talents.

key points to remember as an intermediate-level in Chair Yoga

- ✓ Gradually advance: Accept advancement but avoid rushing into difficult poses or activities. Safety and sustainability are ensured via incremental expansion.
- ✓ Respect Your Boundaries: Recognize your own physical and mental limits. Pushing yourself beyond your limits may result in harm or frustration.
- ✓ Consistent Practice: Consistency is essential. Make regular time to maintain and improve your progress, even if it is for shorter periods of time.
- ✓ Continue to concentrate on your breathing. Breathing in sync with movement deepens postures and promotes mindfulness.

✓ Variation and exploration: Experiment with different styles, positions, and approaches. Diversity in practice makes it interesting and promotes overall improvement.

✓ Seek Help When Needed: If you're having trouble or want to improve, seek help from experienced teachers or trusted resources.

✓ Accept New Challenges: Be willing to try new, more difficult positions or sequences. These obstacles promote growth and resilience.

✓ Balance Strength and Flexibility: For a well-rounded practice, strike a balance between strength-building postures and flexibility-enhancing techniques.

✓ Pay Attention to Your Body: Be aware of your body's cues. Respect any pain or symptoms of strain, and adapt or relax as needed.

✓ Mind-Body link: Increase your understanding of the mind-body link. Take note of how your practice affects your mental and emotional well-being.

✓ Patience and Acceptance: Progress might differ from day to day. Accept swings and setbacks as a natural part of the process.

✓ Reflect and be grateful: Take time to reflect on your progress and be thankful for your journey. Celebrate minor successes and major achievements.

✓ Keep an open mind and a curious mind: Yoga is a broad discipline. In your practice, embrace curiosity by always learning and improving.

✓ Rest and Recovery: Schedule rest days and relaxation exercises to give your body and mind time to recuperate and revitalize.

✓ Community and Support: Participate in the yoga community by seeking support, sharing experiences, and learning from the travels of others.

✓ Take in the scenery: Above all, appreciate the adventure. Create a joyful and fulfilling experience by finding delight in the exercise.

Chapter 6: Chair Yoga Journey (Advanced Level) for 25 Days

Welcome to an energizing 25-day Chair Yoga experience designed specifically for advanced practitioners. This curriculum has been painstakingly designed to increase your practice by focusing on posture correction, mobility enhancement, heart health, and weight control. Accept these advanced-level postures and practices to strengthen your mind-body connection and improve your overall well-being.

Day 1-5: Posture Improvement

Day 1: Advanced Seated Mountain Pose (Tadasana Variation)

- Deepen sitting mountain position by concentrating on grounding, activating core muscles, and lengthening the spine even further.

Day 2: Progression of Seated Backbends

- Investigate advanced sitting backbends that engage core muscles, expand the chest, and increase spinal flexibility.

Day 3: Seated Extended Forward Folds

- Increase the intensity of forward folds by reaching further towards the floor or shins, improving hamstring flexibility and spinal extension.

Day 4: Seated Side Bend Variations:

- Explore complicated sitting side bends, focusing on lateral flexibility and deeper stretches across the sides of the body.

Day 5: Posture Flow for the Entire Body

- Combine skilled posture correction postures into a full sequence that effortlessly integrates breath and movement.

Days 6–10: Mobility Mastery

Day 6: Advanced Knee-to-Chest Stretches

- Deeper knee-to-chest stretches can help with hip flexibility and lower back stretching.

Day 7: Extended Seated Leg Extensions

- Improve your sitting leg extensions by targeting deeper hamstring stretches and keeping appropriate alignment.

Day 8: Warrior Pose Series in a Chair

- Engage in a sequence of advanced warrior postures with chair support to improve lower body strength and stability.

Day 9: Seated Boat Pose Challenge

- Explore advanced sitting boat position variants to engage core muscles and find balance in difficult poses.

Day 10: Chair Supported Camel Pose Progression

- Advance in chair-supported camel postures, deeply opening the front body and increasing spinal flexibility.

Day 11-15: Cardiovascular Health and Stamina

Day 11: Advanced Chair-Supported Heart Openers

- Deeper heart-opening postures with chair support might help with emotional release and circulation.

Day 12: Dynamic Seated Side Bend Stretches

- Engage in dynamic sitting side bend variations, enhancing lateral stretches and encouraging deep breathing.

Day 13: Chair-Supported Forward Bend Twists

- Deeper twists stimulate digestion and improve spine health as you progress in chair-supported forward bend twists.

Day 14: Seated Warrior Pose Fusion

- Dynamically sequence sitting warrior postures to build lower-body strength, stability, and endurance.

Day 15: Standing Pose Flow with a Chair

- Integrate chair-supported standing postures into a flowing flow to improve balance and stamina.

Days 16-20: Weight Management and Core Strengthening

Day 16: Chair-Supported Core Strengthening Intensive

- Concentrate on chair-supported core workouts that target abdominal muscles and promote weight control.

Day 17: Deep Seated Twist and Reach Progression

- Improve oblique engagement and spinal mobility with sitting twist and reach exercises.

Day 18: Chair-Supported Leg Lifts Variations

- Incorporate a variety of chair-supported leg raises to increase lower body strength and stability.

Day 19: Challenging Seated Balance Poses Series

- Sequence difficult sitting balance postures while bearing weight on the chair, developing stability and attention.

Day 20: Chair-Supported High-Intensity Interval Training (HIIT)

- Introduce chair-supported HIIT activities for cardiovascular benefits, including bursts of action and rest periods.

Days 21-25: Integration and Mastery

Day 21: Advanced Chair Yoga Flow Sequence

- Create a complex chair yoga flow by combining advanced positions in a smooth sequence with focused breathing.

Day 22: Chair-Supported Inversions and Extensions

- Investigate chair-supported inversions and extensions, progressively increasing your strength and flexibility in inverted positions.

Day 23: Advanced Chair-Supported Backbends

- Chair-supported backbends are improved, with an emphasis on spinal flexibility and heart-opening feelings.

Day 24: Chair-Supported Forward Folds with Twists

- Deepen chair-supported forward folds with twists to promote purification and rejuvenation.

Day 25: Flow of Mastery and Reflection

- Make a mastery flow sequence that incorporates all mastered postures while also celebrating success and reflecting on the transforming process.

Navigating the 25-Day Advanced-Level Yoga Challenge

Welcome to a thrilling 25-day advanced-level yoga adventure. This program is designed for practitioners who want to enhance their practice by exploring advanced yoga principles and performing challenging postures. Every day is an opportunity to test limits, gain expertise, and undergo metamorphosis.

Day 1-5: Advanced Posture Alignment

Day 1: Advanced Seated Mountain Pose (Tadasana Variation)

- Deepen your practice of sitting mountain position by concentrating on spinal alignment, grounding, and improved breath integration.

Day 2: Advanced Extended Side Angle Pose (Utthita Parsvakonasana) .

- Investigate various versions of the extended side angle stance, focusing on expanded reach and spine elongation.

Day 3: Advanced Chair-Supported Tree Pose (Vrksasana)

- Advanced chair-supported tree poses tests balance while improving alignment and developing the mind-body connection.

Day 4: Extended Seated Bound Angle Pose (Baddha Konasana)

- Improve your sitting bound angle position with advanced variants, concentrating on hip opening and alignment.

Day 5: Full Body Posture Mastery Flow

- Integrate perfected posture alignment postures into a fluid flow, delicately matching breath and movement.

Days 6-10: Fusion of Strength and Flexibility

Day 6: Fusion of Advanced Chair-Supported Warrior Poses

- Sequence warrior postures with chair support to increase strength, stability, and alignment.

Day 7: Advanced Seated Split Pose (Hanumanasana) Exploration

- Work on sitting split pose variations to increase flexibility and stability through advanced adjustments.

Day 8: Advanced Chair-Supported Crow Pose (Bakasana) Progression

- Experiment with crow posture variations while utilizing a chair to help with balance and core activation.

Day 9: Chair Supported Deep Backbends Series

- Dive into advanced backbends while supported by a chair, concentrating on heart opening and spinal flexibility.

Day 10: Dynamic Strength and Flexibility Flow of Fusion

- Incorporate strength-building postures and flexibility sequences into a dynamic flow to promote endurance and flexibility.

Day 11-15: Advanced Balance and Inversions

Day 11: Advanced Chair-Supported Half Moon Pose (Ardha Chandrasana)

- Investigate half-moon position variations with the chair for stability, balance, and open hip engagement.

Day 12: Advanced Inverted Chair Poses series

- Explore advanced inverted postures with the chair, emphasizing controlled inversions and spinal elongation.

Day 13: Fusion of Seated Balancing Poses

- Advanced sitting balancing postures are sequenced, improving attention and stability while perfecting alignment.

Day 14: Preparation for Advanced Chair-Supported Handstands

- Work on handstand preparations using a chair, strengthening the upper body and core in preparation for inversion mastery.

Day 15: Flowing Balance and Inversion Sequences

- Incorporate breath and stability into a fluid sequence of skilled balancing and inversion positions.

Days 16-20: Advanced Pranayama and Meditation

Day 16: Advanced Pranayama (Kapalabhati, Bhastrika) Practice

- Explore advanced pranayama methods, emphasizing regulated breathing and interior purification.

Day 17: Preparation for Advanced Chair-Supported Lotus Pose (Padmasana)

- Work on lotus position preparations in the chair, promoting hip flexibility and attentive meditation preparation.

Day 18:Extended Meditation Practices

- Through seated and reclined positions, experiment with extended periods of meditation, refining attention and inner awareness.

Day 19: Advanced Chair-Supported Prone Poses (Makarasana)

- Prone positions with chair support promote relaxation and attentive grounding.

Day 20: Integration of Flowing Pranayama and Meditation

- Integrate advanced pranayama and meditation techniques into a unified flow that promotes harmony and inner calm.

Day 21-25: Culmination and Mastery

Day 21: Integration of the Mastery Flow

- Create a thorough flow that incorporates mastered postures while also celebrating progress and reflecting on the trip.

Day 22: Advanced Chair-Supported Backbends and Twists

- Using chair support, deepen backbends and twists, improving spinal flexibility and detoxifying.

Day 23: Advanced Chair-Supported Forward Folds (Paschimottanasana)

- Refine forward folds with chair support, focusing on elongation and relaxation across the back body.

Day 24: Advanced Chair Yoga Flow Series

- Arrange advanced postures in a flowing series to demonstrate mastery and fluidity in transitions.

Day 25: Mastery Reflection and Celebration

- Celebrate the challenge's completion with a reflection session that recognizes accomplishments and emerging talents.

key points to remember as an advanced-level in Chair Yoga

✓ Caution is advised before progressing to the advanced level. Push the boundaries gradually to avoid damage or strain.

✓ Mindful Mastery: Concentrate on improving alignment, breathing, and mental attention in difficult postures. When it comes to yoga (and many other things), it's more about how well you practice rather than how much you do. Quality beats quantity.

✓ To guarantee safe and successful practice, seek expert help from experienced teachers for difficult postures or methods.

✓ Stability and adaptability Maintain a balance of strength-building and flexibility-enhancing routines for a well-rounded practice.

✓ Take Care of Your Body: Pay close attention to your body's cues. Recognize your limitations and honor your body's demand for rest or adaptation.

✓ Mind-Body Connection: Increase the depth of your mind-body connection. In advanced postures, embrace the interaction of breath, movement, and mental attention.

✓ Challenge yourself on a regular basis without growing complacent. Continuous development promotes the progress of your profession.

✓ Introspection and adaptation: Review your practice on a regular basis. Adapt and improve strategies based on your observations and observations.

✓ Perseverance and patience are required since advanced postures can be difficult to learn. Persist despite difficulties; realizing improvement may be sluggish.

✓ Approach your practice with humility and openness. Maintain an open mind to learning and perfecting even the most fundamental components of yoga.

✓ Rest and Recovery: Maintain a healthy balance of intensity and rest. In order to preserve physical and emotional well-being, incorporate recovery methods.

✓ Celebrate Progress: Recognize and celebrate achievements in your advanced practice. Celebrate the trip as well as the goal.

✓ Injury Prevention: Make safety and injury prevention a top priority. Recognize your body's limitations and avoid pushing it beyond its capabilities.

✓ Mental Resilience: Develop your mental resilience and flexibility by learning from your setbacks and obstacles on your advanced path.

✓ Sharing and Community: Within the yoga community, share your views and experiences. Participate in conversations and learn from the advanced practices of others.

Chapter 7: Chair Yoga Meets Meditation

What's mediation

Meditation is a mental activity that involves training attention and awareness in order to gain mental clarity, emotional quiet, and deep inner peace. It is a practice with ancient roots that may be found in diverse forms throughout countries, faiths, and philosophies.

Meditation is, at its core, an intentional and concentrated practice aimed at quieting the mind, cultivating awareness, and promoting a sense of inner peace. Contrary to common assumption, it is about witnessing ideas, sensations, and emotions without judgment rather than repressing or emptying the mind.

Mindfulness, breath awareness, loving-kindness, transcendental meditation, and body scan meditation are just a few examples of meditation approaches. Each approach has its own methodologies, but they all aim to cultivate present-moment mindfulness and mental calm.

Meditation, in essence, provides a space for people to halt, examine their thoughts without attachment, and connect with their inner selves. Individuals may feel lower stress, increased attention and concentration, improved emotional control, and a greater sense of self-awareness and well-being via frequent practice.

Meditation may be done anywhere, from tranquil meditation facilities to the comfort of one's own home. Assuming a comfortable position, focusing attention on a selected object (such as the breath, a mantra, or physiological sensations), and gently redirecting attention anytime the mind wanders are common practices.

general, meditation is an effective technique for mental, emotional, and spiritual development, building a better awareness of oneself and the world, and increasing general well-being.

Profound Benefits of combining chair yoga and meditation.

Combining chair yoga with meditation techniques provides a transforming journey that goes beyond physical exercise and mental relaxation, diving into a realm of comprehensive well-being, inner serenity, and profound self-discovery. The combination of these disciplines produces a synergy that magnifies their individual advantages, raising one's mental, emotional, and physical health to new heights.

Chair Yoga as a Route to Mindful Movement

Chair yoga, which evolved from conventional yoga principals, makes the ancient practice accessible to everyone, regardless of age, mobility, or physical restrictions. It combines modified yoga positions, breathwork, and meditation practices, all of which are done while sitting or supported by a chair.

Enhanced Flexibility and Mobility: Gentle stretches and motions enhance joint flexibility and mobility, reducing stiffness and pain.

Improved Posture: A focus on alignment aids in the cultivation of improved posture, decreasing strain and tension in the body.

Mindful movement and breathwork soothe the nervous system, relieving tension and increasing relaxation.

Improved Circulation: Movement sequences increase blood flow, which improves circulation and general vigor.

Mind-Body Connection: Chair yoga promotes a stronger bond between the mind and the body, increasing self-awareness and mindfulness.

Meditation's Importance in Chair Yoga

Meditation, which is frequently incorporated into chair yoga sessions, acts as a potent complement, multiplying the benefits of the practice. While chair yoga focuses on physical well-being, meditation focuses inward, cultivating mental clarity and emotional balance.

Mindfulness Amplification: Meditation expands on the mindfulness developed via chair yoga, developing greater awareness of thoughts and sensations.

Emotional Regulation: Regular chair yoga meditation practice helps with emotion management, lowering reactivity, and increasing emotional resilience.

Stress Reduction and Relaxation: Meditation techniques included into chair yoga sessions promote profound relaxation, stress relief, and a sense of tranquility.

Enhanced Mental attention: Chair yoga practitioners sharpen their attention and concentration via meditation, improving mental clarity and cognitive performance.

Chair Yoga and Meditation Work Together

When chair yoga and meditation are combined, they produce a harmonic synergy that feeds both the body and the mind. Chair yoga warms up the body by releasing tension and increasing flexibility, whilst meditation sharpens mental attention and inner awareness. This mutually beneficial connection promotes a comprehensive approach to well-being that includes physical health, mental clarity, emotional balance, and spiritual progress.

Creating Mind-Body Balance

Chair yoga's mild motions complement meditation, promoting a balanced flow of energy throughout the body.

Inner calm and Tranquility: Chair yoga incorporates meditation, which promotes inner calm and tranquillity even while moving.

Increased Self-Awareness: The combination increases self-awareness, allowing practitioners to delve deeper into the mind-body link.

Techniques for Integrating Meditation into Chair Yoga Image Suggestion: Chair yoga poses demonstrated in conjunction with meditation postures and quiet environs.

Incorporate mindful breathing techniques into chair yoga, concentrating on the inhalation and exhalation rhythm.

Visualization: During chair yoga sequences, guide practitioners through visualizations to promote relaxation and inner peace.

Body Scan Meditation: Use body scan techniques to encourage awareness of bodily sensations during times of quiet in chair yoga.

Silent Meditation: Set aside time during chair yoga sessions for silent meditation, allowing practitioners to explore inner calm.

Realizing the Potential for Change

The combination of chair yoga and meditation unleashes transforming potential, providing practitioners with a holistic approach to well-being. Individuals go on a journey of self-discovery, empowerment, and holistic healing by combining movement, breath, and mindfulness.

Basic Meditation poses and practices for beginners:

1. *Sukhasana (Easy Pose) Seated Meditation*

- Posture: Sit comfortably on a chair or cushion with your legs crossed and your spine upright yet relaxed. Hands can be placed on the knees or in any comfortable posture.
- Focus: Gently close your eyes or cast a gentle glance ahead. Bring your focus to the natural movement of your breath, naturally inhaling and exhaling.
- Technique: Concentrate on your breath, watching its rhythm. As ideas come, recognize them without judgment before gently returning your attention to your breathing.

2. Body Scan Meditation

- Posture: Lie comfortably on your back with your legs outstretched and your arms at your sides, palms facing upward.
- Focus: Start with your toes and progressively extend your attention to each region of your body, feeling sensations of tightness.
- Technique: Consciously relax each bodily part. Breathe deeply into any tense places, allowing them to dissipate as you exhale.

3. Mindful Walking Meditation

- Posture: Locate a peaceful area. Begin slowly and gradually, at a comfortable pace.
- Focus: Pay attention to each stride, noticing how your foot lifts, goes forward, and hits the ground.
- Technique: Engage all of your senses by noticing the movement of your body, the noises around you, and the sensation of air against your skin.

4. Mantra Meditation

- Posture: Sit on a chair or on the floor comfortably, with your eyes closed or lightly focused.

- Focus: Choose a word, phrase, or sound to repeat quietly or softly aloud (mantra).

- Technique: Repeat the mantra with each breath, synchronizing the sound or word with the inhale and expiration.

5. Relaxation Meditation

- Posture: Sit comfortably with your eyes closed and take a few deep breaths.

- Focus: Imagine a peaceful area or setting, such as a beach, forest, or other relaxing environment.

- Technique: Involve all of your senses in the visualization – feel the temperature, smell the fragrances, and imagine the surroundings clearly.

Beginners' Tips:

- ✓ Start with small workouts (5-10 minutes) and progressively increase as you get more comfortable.

✓ Find a peaceful, comfortable place where you will not be bothered.

✓ Patience: Be gentle with yourself; it's natural for your mind to wander. Return your attention to the technique you've chosen.

✓ Guided Meditation: To supplement your practice, consider using guided meditation apps or CDs.

Advanced Meditation Practices and Their Integration

Meditation, which is frequently seen as a timeless practice founded in ancient wisdom, emerges in a variety of forms, each of which offers a distinct route to self-discovery, heightened awareness, and inner tranquillity. As practitioners progress farther along their meditation path, advanced techniques develop, providing great chances for spiritual growth, expanded consciousness, and a deeper connection with the self and the cosmos.

Advanced Meditation Methods

1. *Vipassana (Insight Meditation) Meditation*

- Vipassana meditation focuses on examining body sensations, thoughts, and emotions with strong awareness, free of attachment or judgment.
- Practitioners monitor sensations throughout the body, scanning from head to toe or vice versa, building mindfulness and insight into the impermanence of experiences.

2. Meditation Metta (Loving-Kindness)

- Metta meditation fosters sentiments of love, compassion, and goodwill toward oneself, loved ones, neutral people, and even problematic people.
- Practitioners repeat loving–kindness mantras, focusing positive thoughts towards themselves and others, cultivating empathy and compassion.

3. Transcendental Meditation (TM)

- Focus: TM entails quietly repeating a certain mantra, which allows the mind to transcend ideas and achieve a state of deep relaxation and heightened awareness.
- A certified instructor initiates practitioners into TM, providing them with a customized mantra to utilize during meditation sessions.

4. *Kundalini Meditation:*

- Kundalini meditation seeks to awaken the latent energy (kundalini) in the base of the spine, promoting spiritual enlightenment and self-realization.
- Technique: Practitioners channel energy along the chakras by using breathwork (pranayama), chanting, and certain body movements (kriyas).

Advanced Meditation in Your Practice

The incorporation of advanced meditation methods necessitates a methodical and deliberate approach. Incorporating these approaches into a daily meditation practice can help to deepen the practice and reveal new levels of self-awareness and spiritual progress.

Progressive Development:

- Consistency: Begin by progressively incorporating advanced methods into existing meditation sessions.
- Extended Sessions: Gradually increase the duration of meditation to suit advanced practices, providing for more time for in-depth inquiry.

Mindset and Environment

- Sacred place: Create a calm setting favorable to advanced practices, such as a quiet, devoted meditation place
- Approach advanced approaches with an open and receptive mentality, appreciating the adventure with no expectations.

Support and guided instruction

- Seek expert advice from experienced teachers or websites specializing in advanced meditation methods.
- Community and Support: Join meditation communities or organizations to exchange experiences and get help on your advanced meditation journey.

Practical tips on infusing meditation into daily routines.

Certainly, adding meditation into everyday activities enables people to reap the advantages of mindfulness, improving well-being in the face of life's pressures. Here are some helpful hints for incorporating meditation into your daily life:

1. Morning Routines

- Early Morning: Get up a few minutes early to devote time to meditation before the day begins.
- Begin the day with a brief meditation practice to create a pleasant tone for the day ahead.

- Focus Techniques: To match with the day's aims and ambitions, try breath-focused or intention-setting meditations.

2. Mindful Moments

- Micro-Meditations: Take brief breaks (even just a minute or two) during the day to practice mini-meditation sessions, concentrating on breath or sensations.
- Incorporate Mindfulness into Routine tasks: Incorporate mindfulness into routine tasks such as cleaning dishes, strolling, or sipping tea by concentrating on the present moment sensations.

3. Workday Integration

- Lunchtime Reset: Use your lunch breaks to meditate for a few minutes, refreshing your mind for the afternoon ahead.
- Desk Meditation: Take a few moments at your desk to practice mindful breathing or gentle

stretching to renew your attention and relieve tension.

4. Evening Relaxation

- Post-work Transition: Decompress from the workday by engaging in a meditation practice before switching to personal time.
- Relaxation Techniques: Use meditation before bedtime to wind down and promote relaxation for a pleasant night's sleep.

5. Creating a Ritual

- Designate an area: Create a specific meditation area at home, such as a quiet nook or a room devoid of distractions.
- Set definite periods for meditation every day, creating a ritual that becomes an intrinsic part of the habit.

6. Technology as an Aid

- Guided Sessions: Look into meditation apps or online resources that provide guided meditation sessions customized to different time limits and goals.

- Reminder applications: For scheduled meditation sessions, use smartphone applications with reminders or timers.

7. Integration of Mindfulness

- Mindful Eating: During meals, practice mindfulness by enjoying each mouthful and concentrating on sensory stimuli.
- Integrate meditation with activities such as yoga, tai chi, or walking, stressing present moment awareness.us

Important Point for Mediation

1. Regularity and consistency

- ✓ Commitment: Set aside a consistent amount of time each day for meditation, even if it is only a few minutes.
- ✓ Create a meditation habit that is a non-negotiable element of your daily agenda.

2. Relaxed Posture Alignment:

- ✓ Sit or lie comfortably, keeping your spine straight yet relaxed to allow for effortless breathing.
- ✓ Position: Find a comfortable position for yourself, whether sat on a cushion, on a chair, or lying down.

3. Breath Control

- ✓ Focused Breathing: To create attention and tranquility, utilize the breath as an anchor, monitoring its natural rhythm.
- ✓ Observe the sensation of the breath without attempting to regulate it.

4. Non-Judgment Observation

- ✓ Mindful Awareness: Without judgment or attachment, observe ideas, feelings, and emotions as they emerge.

✓ Allowing ideas to Pass: Allow ideas to pass through before restoring concentration to the breath or selected place of focus.

5. Acceptance and Patience

✓ Understand that the mind will stray; gently direct it back to the present without self-criticism.

✓ Acceptance: Accept each meditation session for what it is, without anticipating specific results.

6. Gradual Improvement

✓ Begin with shorter sessions and progressively increase the time as your practice develops.

✓ Recognize that growth in meditation comes from persistent practice over time.

7. Curiosity and openness

✓ Approach meditation with curiosity, experimenting with various techniques and approaches.

✓ Open Heart: Develop an open and receptive mentality, enabling events to organically emerge.

8. Guided Assistance

✓ Guided Sessions: Think about utilizing guided meditations or apps to help you with your practice.

✓ Seek advice from experienced teachers or organizations for a better understanding.

9. Compassion and gratitude

✓ Grateful Mindset: Begin and conclude sessions with gratitude to promote a happy attitude.

✓ Self-Compassion: Show yourself kindness during the exercise; it's alright to have wandering thoughts.

10. Integration into Everyday Life

✓ Mindful Living: Incorporate meditation ideas into daily activities by practicing awareness in ordinary chores.

✓ Consistent Effort: Keep in mind that meditation is
a lifetime adventure with advantages that extend
beyond the practice.

Conclusion

Certainly! As your chair yoga adventure comes to an end, it's important to consider the transforming potential and long-term influence of this practice on your well-being. This epilogue represents both a conclusion and a new beginning, with the confluence of your experiences laying the groundwork for future growth, health, and balance.

Reflecting on the Impact of Chair Yoga at the End of Your Journey

You've spent the last 25 days exploring mindful movement, breath, and inner discovery via chair yoga. Take a minute to appreciate the progress you've made, the insights you've acquired, and the physical and mental improvements you've observed. Chair yoga is more than simply a set of postures; it's a journey of self-discovery that promotes better posture, flexibility, and a stronger mind-body connection.

Continuing Practice: Chair Yoga and Meditation

As this chapter comes to a close, it's vital to remember that your chair yoga and meditation journey is one that should be continued and integrated into your everyday life. Accept the empowerment and vigor that chair yoga has given you. Use these resources to help you handle life's obstacles, discover moments of quiet in the midst of stress, and cultivate a deeper sense of well-being.

Final Thoughts: Maintaining a Balanced, Healthier Lifestyle

In closing, keep in mind that your road toward a better living is multifaceted and includes more than just chair yoga. Continue to emphasize self-care, feeding both the body and the mind. Incorporate healthy habits into your daily routine, such as mindful eating, frequent exercising, and times of meditation. Adopt a balanced way of living that promotes your physical, emotional, and spiritual well-being.

This epilogue signals the beginning of a new chapter in your wellness journey, not the conclusion. As you finish your chair yoga practice, remember the lessons you learned, the strength you acquired, and the peace you encountered. Accept change as an ever-present companion on your journey to a better and more satisfying life.

Last Thoughts: Your Health, Your Story

Remember that the core of your tale is in your hands while you pursue happiness. Chair yoga and meditation have built the framework, providing self-care and resilience techniques. Seize each day with purpose, enjoying life's fullness and nurturing your body, mind, and soul.

THANK

YOU